NATURAL REMEDIES

NATURAL REMEDIES

A Step-By-Step Guide to Making and Using Herbal Medicines

María Tránsito López Luengo
and Carlota Máñez Arisó

Translated by Gladis Beatriz Castillo

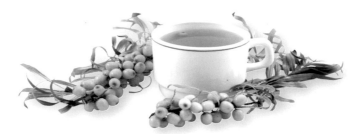

Skyhorse Publishing

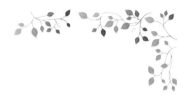

For those who know that the secret to good health lies in small but valuable practices.

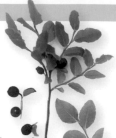

Contents

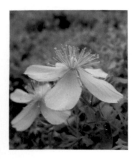

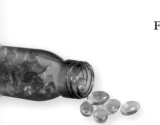

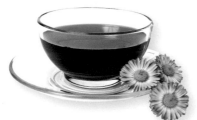

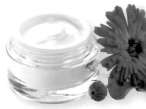

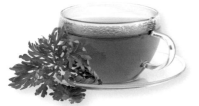

Introduction

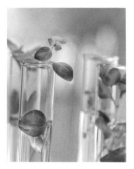

Until recently, if you take into account the slow development of therapeutic treatments, plants have been the major source of cures against disease and human suffering. Historically, medicinal plants have been inextricably tied to the progress of medicine and the pharmaceutical profession. The discovery of the New World also led to the discovery of new therapeutic possibilities that made Spain the center of development for herbal medicine in the sixteenth century, which later spread to other European countries. However, the isolation of morphine from opium in the early nineteenth century led to the isolation of many other active ingredients, which set off the current and unstoppable development of synthetic chemistry and the continued devaluation of herbal medicine. This decline in the use of medicinal plants can be attributed, first of all, to the numerous synthetic drugs that were successful in eradicating various diseases for which medicinal plants were not effective. For example, sulfonamides, then antibiotics (which are also of plant origin), led us to change word break to be-lieve that we had managed to overcome disease, but new diseases, degenerative conditions, and disorders related to a sedentary lifestyle and increased life expectancy emerged.

It was then that the side effects of synthetic drugs started to become known, and this awareness forced us into creating standards of safety and efficacy that are critical for any substance for which medicinal claims are made.

Our new economic organization has been one of the biggest barriers against using medicinal plants. The development of patents and trademarks is one of the main reasons natural medicines are not more widely used, because they are unpatentable, and herbal medicine in particular has often been relegated to developing countries that lack economic resources. Indeed, although herbal medicine is one of the oldest and most wide-spread practices, orthodox medicine has neglected it, and the use of herbs today is restricted to those who opt for alternative medicine, taking a holistic view of the body that aims to treat people, not illnesses, in a manner that is consistent with natural laws. In comparison to using drugs that only relieve symptoms and often have side effects, herbal medicine promotes using medicinal plants to help recover our overall health and maintain it.

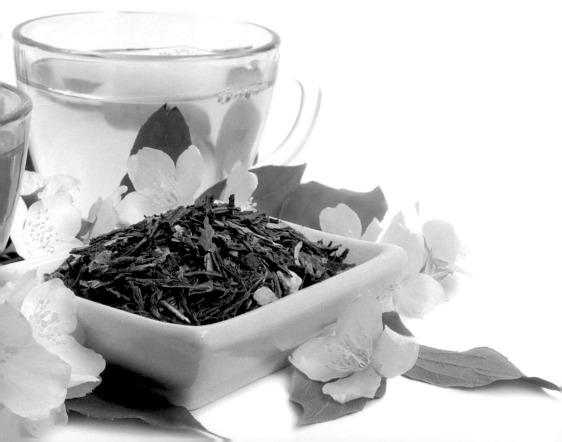

Plants for health and wellness

Fortunately, nowadays, it seems that we are witnessing a resurgence of natural therapies, and we can even say that the pharmaceutical market for medicinal plant products is booming again after a long period in which it was overshadowed by synthetic drugs and biotech. Among other factors, this resurgence is due to the growing interest in natural products, wider knowledge of the pharmacological properties of plants, and greater safety concerns regarding many synthetic drugs. Indeed, since the seventies, there has been a growing interest in herbal medicine at a grassroots level as well as in research labs. One factor that has led to this renewed appeal of medicinal plants is the belief that everything natural is good. However, this belief is misleading; just because a product is touted as being natural, it is not necessarily going to have better quality or safety. Oftentimes people believe that the benefits of herbal medicine far outweigh the artificiality of synthetic drugs, but this is choosing to ignore the fact that there are many toxic plants and that most drugs used in conventional medicine have active ingredients that derive from plants.

On the other hand, interest in medicinal plants does not exist only at the grassroots level. There are other factors in the scientific field that are pushing for herbal medicine to become again a branch of therapeutics. Both scientific development, which allows us to better understand their pharmacological properties, and the current ability to prepare dosage forms with active ingredients, which enable a consistent preparation ensuring guarantees of quality, efficacy, and safety, play a decisive role in the reassessment of medicinal plant based products. Health professionals, doctors, and pharmacists have also become more aware of less aggressive medications, such as herbal medicine, which has slower reaction times and fewer side effects, which in most cases are mild and temporary.

In recent years, as a result of this resurgence of medicinal plants as effective and safe therapeutic alternatives, the market for products derived from plants is seeing a major upward trend, not only in our country but also in other countries within the European Community. Specifically, in 2006, there were a total of 1,110 different products with medicinal plants registered in the database of the General Council of Official Colleges of Pharmacists. Of these, products with plant laxatives are the most abundant in pharmacies. Often this group includes anti-obesity preparations that are used in weight loss treatments. Secondly, they include plants for treating insomnia and other symptoms associated with anxiety. The top-selling third group is made up of digestive plants, including carminative, antispasmodic, and stimulating species that help intestinal digestion. This group usually includes phytotherapeutic products that stimulate the production of bile, which are used to improve symptoms of biliary dyspepsia. Finally, there are herbal preparations for cardiovascular health, especially those that have anti-hypertensive and venotonic effects.

This book was born out of our career paths, as well as many conversations, and our common interest in a more natural way to care for our health. María, a pharmaceutical technician specialized in nutrition and dietetics and expert in medicinal plants, and Carlota, a journalist with extensive experience in health magazines and wellness, are united by the passion to impart all the knowledge we have acquired over many years. Our work has become a lifestyle for us and given us this book, along with another book published by this same publisher (*Natural Health for Women*). Writing these books has given us the opportunity to put into writing, arrange, and investigate one of the issues on which both of us have worked and that has been part of our conversations since the day we met.

Of course, this book is not intended to be an exhaustive treatise on medicinal plants. Our goal was to develop an attractive and engaging guide that brings practical information about the most common medicinal plants in our country. This book aims to become a useful tool for those seeking to support their health and wellbeing with the use of medicinal plants in their daily life (in the bathroom, the kitchen, while traveling . . .). This work is the result of the collection of numerous studies showing the effectiveness and safety of the plants described. We thank Esther Sanz, our editor, for the trust she has given us, and the work of the entire Océano team. The result is obvious, and hopefully it will become a reference book for those who want to take care of themselves in a more natural way that respects people and the environment.

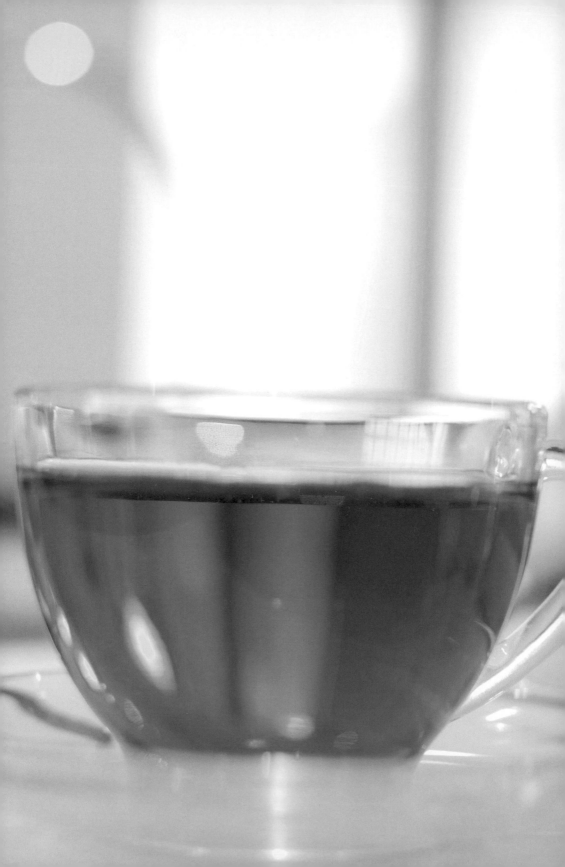

Get to know them

What they do for you

Each day more and more people become acquainted with medicinal plants. Who has not taken a chamomile tea after a hearty meal? Who has not used some linden tea to calm their nerves before bed? Beyond these popular remedies, there is room in your home medicine cabinet for others that have been proven effective to relieve everyday problems and that offer more advantages than synthetic products. Looking at the entire repertoire that nature offers us, it is easy to find plants that have great healing properties and can be very useful to treat many ailments. In fact, of the 50,000 to 70,000 varieties of plants that are estimated to have ever been used for therapeutic purposes, we offer a selection of the most well-known plants that are easy to find in health food stores and pharmacies. Rosemary, thyme, bay, anise, dandelion . . . these are varieties that you have seen more than once in their natural state, and now you will know how to use them at home and discover how they can help against all kinds of disorders.

However, keep in mind that self-medication with herbal remedies is also dangerous; therefore, you must pay attention to the dosage and potential risks.

Why do they heal?

The fact that we can claim that certain plants are "medicinal" means that they possess a number of biologically active substances, active ingredients, which give them the ability to act on certain ailments. Although there are still many components waiting to be discovered, some of them have been identified and isolated, and research has allowed us to better understand their effects on the body. In most cases, the medicinal effect of a given plant depends on not just one but various active ingredients acting synergistically together. Generally, one plant has different properties that are useful in different situations, and it is more efficient to use the plant than to use just one of its active ingredients separately.

Keep in mind that the content of these substances can vary within a species, depending on factors such as irrigation, soil, harvesting time, and so forth. We have grouped the plants into several categories according to their chemical nature. The most important ones are shown in the table below.

The most important active ingredients

● **Carbohydrates**
Also known as saccharide, they are abundant and there are several types. The most significant are:

Sugars: simple carbohydrates (such as glucose and fructose). They have a toning effect and are abundant in fruits.
Mucilage: solution with a gelatinous consistency, often found on the outer integument of seeds, as well as in other organs of the plant. They hold water, swell, and increase in volume, so some plants that are rich in mucilage act as laxatives, to relieve coughing, and to treat skin disorders. Greater plantains, mallow, linden flower, and aloe are rich in mucilage.
Inulin: this complex carbohydrate promotes digestion and is well tolerated by diabetics. Chicory and dandelion are rich in inulin.

● **Lipids**
The most important group of plant-derived fatty substances are oils.

Oils: are obtained by cold pressing the seeds and fruits of several plant species. They usually consist of unsaturated fatty acids and are liquid. They have laxative, lipid lowering (cholesterol lowering), and emollient properties. Evening primrose oil, olive oil, and borage oil are the most common.

● **Amino acids**
Although you can find them in free form, you most often see them as part of more complex structures. The most important are:

Enzymes: although plants have many enzymatic compounds, only some of them such as proteolytic enzymes are used in phytotherapy. A plant that stands out for its content of such enzymes is the papaya.
Sulfur compounds: some plants have a series of active sulfur compounds that are biosynthesized from amino acids. One of the most common is garlic.

● **Phenolic compounds**
Simple phenols: this group includes compounds that are less abundant in nature and have a limited therapeutic value, except for hydroquinone, which is in plants like bear-berry or bearberry and some types of heather.
Coumarins: affect the vascular system, both arterial and venous circulation, and they are also useful for treating certain skin disorders, such as psoriasis. Some of these are horse-chestnut and angelica.
Tannins: for centuries they have been used for their ability to convert skin into leather, as well as for their internal and external astringent properties. Internally, they are used as an anti-diarrheal and vaso-

constrictors. Externally, they are used as vaso-constrictors for certain skin problems, such as dermatosis, and in cosmetics as astringent tonics. They are also antioxidants. Witch-hazel is rich in tannins.
Flavonoids: an important group that is widely distributed in nature, with simple and complex structures. They are often responsible for the coloring of flowers, fruit, and leaves (anthocyanins). They act on the vascular system, strengthening and toning the vein walls. They also have anti-inflammatory and antioxidant effects. Some of the most significant plants containing them are passionflower, ginkgo, milk thistle, and hawthorn.

● **Terpenes**
Essential oils: complex, liquid mixtures that are volatile. In general, they give plants their unique scent and have an antiseptic, antispasmodic, expectorant, carminative, and digestive effect. At high doses, they are toxic, mainly on the central nervous system. Some can cause topical problems, such as irritation and allergies. Some plants with essential oil are chamomile, peppermint, anise, eucalyptus, and clove.
Sesquiterpenes: traditionally, sesquiterpenes have been considered "bitter" substances.

Their main actions are anti-inflammatory, antimicrobial, and appetite stimulating. They include burdock and wormwood.
Triterpenes and steroids: this group includes saponins that have expectorant and diuretic effect, such as licorice root, horse-chestnut, and ginseng root.

● **Alkaloids**
This is a series of complex and very active nitrogen compounds; even in small doses they have a great effect on the body. They are very effective for different conditions, but if you exceed the recommended dose, they can also be poisonous. There are many plants, such as fumitory, that act using alkaloids.

Take them internally

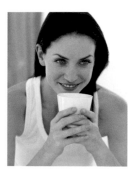

There are multiple ways to extract and apply active plant substances and benefit from their healing properties. The most appropriate method in each case always depends on the plant and the type of condition being treated. They can be administered internally and applied externally. These are the most common forms of internal administration:

Infusion

Infusion is the simplest way to prepare a remedy using the delicate parts of plants, leaves, flowers, tops, and tender stems. To prepare it, all you have to do is add two teaspoons of the plant to two cups of boiling water. Then let it steep for 10 to 15 minutes and strain. You can drink it hot, lukewarm, or even cold if that is what you prefer. Logically, if you are suffering from a cold, you will want to drink it hot. This remedy can be sweetened with honey, other natural sweetener, or apple juice.

Herbal teas

Herbal teas are probably the most popular way to ingest medicinal plants. They are often made through infusion, decoction, or maceration. You can group several plants together to enhance their effect. Teas are primarily used orally, but as you will see throughout this book, you can also use them topically.

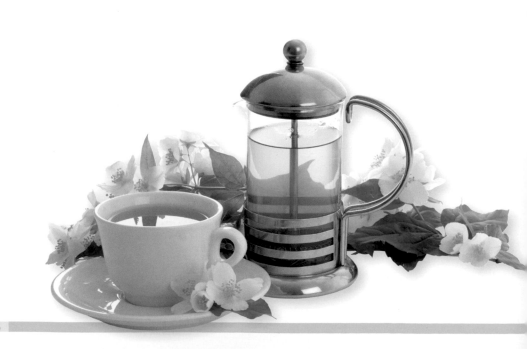

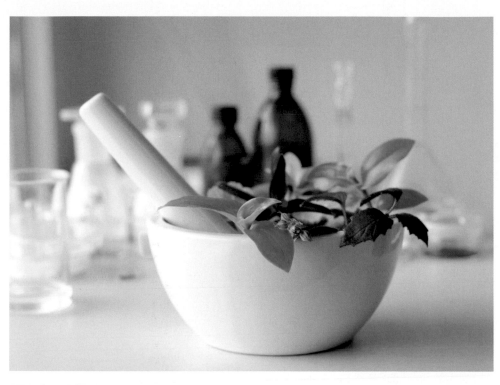

Syrups and potions

To prepare syrups, use simple syrup consisting of water containing 64% sucrose (sugar), and add tinctures or liquid extracts. Syrups are easy and pleasant, and their sweetness masks the bad taste of many plants, which makes it easier to administer to children. Also try using honey instead of sucrose. Potions are similar to syrups but have lower sucrose content.

Juice

Juice is obtained by squeezing the fresh plant. When the plant is too dry or woody, it has to be submerged in hot water. The juice can be ingested or used externally.

Tincture

Tinctures are alcoholic solutions that are prepared by steeping the dried and crushed plant in alcohol at room temperature for two or three days. Alcohol should be suitable for human consumption (never use industrial, denatured, or rubbing alcohol as these are toxic). Dilute them before ingesting (15 to 25 drops in a little water). Due to their alcoholic content, they are contraindicated for individuals suffering from liver disease, pregnant women, children, as well as for people undergoing treatment against alcohol addiction. They can also be used topically.

Powder

Administering in powder form helps you get most of the active ingredients, especially if they are located in the hard parts of the plant (roots, bark, and seeds). Although some people take the powder alone or mix it with food, it is not a very user-friendly method, so take it in capsules or tablets.

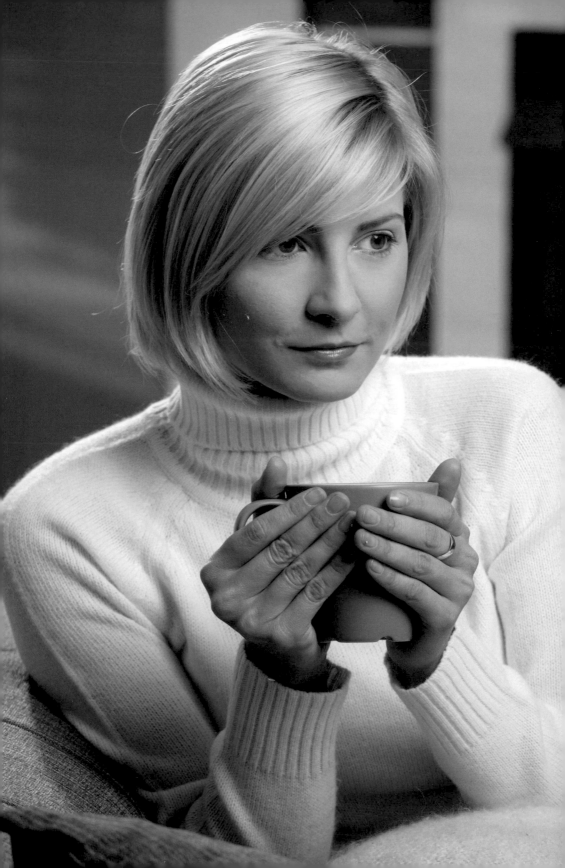

Decoction

The proper amount of the plant is placed in hot water and boiled for 2 to minutes. It is then left to macerate for 15 minutes. The resulting liquid is strained and consumed preferably hot, but it can also be ingested warm or cold. It is used to make herbal teas from the hard parts of plants (roots, bark, seeds), which require sustained boiling to release their active ingredients.

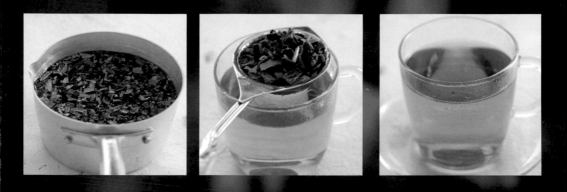

Maceration

The plant is placed in an opaque container with the required amount of water at room temperature in a cool, dark place for a certain amount of time, and then the resulting liquid is strained. Generally, the soaking period for delicate parts is about 12 hours, and for the hard parts it is 24 hours. This method is very useful for plants whose active ingredients are thermolabile (altered by heat).

Some plants may also be macerated in oil, to be used externally. This preparation should not be confused with extracting its essential oil, which is an active ingredient of the plant itself. Once prepared, they are to be kept in frosted glass containers to avoid losing their effectiveness.

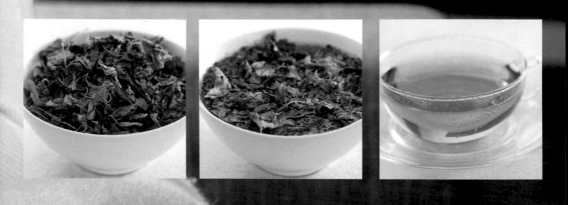

Apply them externally

Creams or ointments

Semisolid forms that are generally made up of an emulsified mixture of water and fat or oil. They are applied directly on the skin or mucous membranes, and their active ingredients are used during the preparation process.

Baths

To prepare them, simply add an infusion or decoction (at least 1.5 quart (1.5 liter) of the plant to your bathwater, or you can also dilute 2 to 5 drops of essential oil into bathwater. This method of administration is particularly useful for relieving aching limbs, inflammation, rheumatic pain, and nasal congestion.

The bath can be for the whole body or for the feet, hands, and eyes.

Plasters and poultices

Plasters and poultices consist of applying fresh, dried, or cooked herbs directly on the affected area. They can be applied hot or cold, with a cloth or gauze, or directly after applying oil on the affected area so as to prevent the plant mixture from sticking. Leave on for 5 to 10 minutes; it is better to use several short applications throughout the day rather than a single and prolonged one.

Compresses

Compresses are easier to use than poultices, although their effect is less intense. Moisten a piece of cloth with a few drops of essential oil dissolved in water, an infusion, or decoction or fresh juice, and then apply it (preferably hot) on the affected area for 5 to 10 minutes, depending on the plant.

Vapor

Place the plants or selected essential oil into a container and add boiling water. Then cover your head with a towel and inhale the steam for 20 minutes, eyes closed, trying to breathe normally until it cools off. It is great for clearing your respiratory tract.

Mouth rinses

They can be done with an infusion, decoction, or diluted tincture (1 teaspoon (5 ml) of tincture per ½ cup (100 ml) of water). Do not use very hot or very concentrated liquids, and do not swallow it. They are useful for alleviating conditions of the mouth and throat.

Precautions

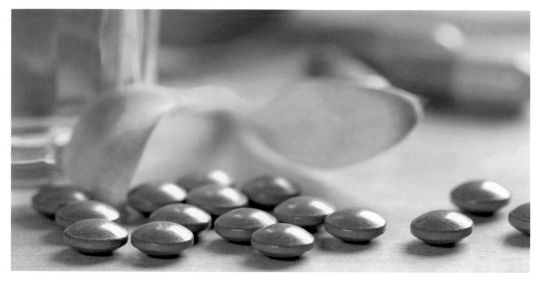

In recent years, there has been growing use of medicinal plants in combination with other conventional medicines. However, keep in mind that self-diagnosing and self-medicating is generally not recommended because although most plants are safe, they are not always harmless. Just as they are likely to improve your health, their misuse or improper combination may have adverse effects and negative interactions with other medications. Many plants have very potent active ingredients, so it is best to consult with a specialist who can recommend adequate treatment and proper dosage.

Side effects and interactions

Medicinal plants work like medications since their therapeutic effect is attributed to their pharmacologically active agents. For this reason, they may cause side effects, mainly due to inadvertent use of the wrong plant species, alteration of the plant, or an overdose. Similarly, drug interactions may occur due to simultaneously administering them with other allopathic medicines.

Responsible use

Although most common plants are harmless, before using them you should be aware that some of them have adverse side effects and negative interactions when combined with certain medications.

Most interactions may lessen or increase the effects of the drug and even cause serious problems. Having the right information helps prevent many problems.

Contraindications

Given that certain medicinal plants can cause negative side effects and interactions, they may be contraindicated in certain situations, so it is important to seek good professional advice before taking any herbal remedy. There are physiological situations where contra-indications are more common, such as during pregnancy and lactation. In such cases, using plants that have some level of toxicity is contraindicated. Often, because there is not enough research that ensures complete safety, it is also advised that pregnant and nursing women avoid even those plants that could be considered safe. Children and older adults are two delicate age groups with whom you must take extra precautions.

Where to buy them

Health food shops are where people typically get medicinal plants in their most varied forms: dry, fresh, powder, tincture, and others. And it is where you can buy a wider variety of remedies of this kind. The herbalist is usually skilled and knowledgeable and can answer questions about any particular remedy. Although many shops are family-owned and handed down from generation to generation, their products are also subject to appropriate quality controls. In Spain, you can also buy herbal medicines in pharmacies, an option that more and more people resort to since they offer the same guarantees as with synthetic drugs, that is, health records, and this gives consumers peace of mind. This health record is unique to pharmacological preparations sold in pharmacies, and it certifies that a drug, whether synthetic or plant-based, exceeded efficacy and safety controls established by the Ministry of Health. Products sold in pharmacies are packaged and distributed by the manufacturers, so it is easier to find them in drugstores, phytotherapy treatment centers, and health stores. An important difference with the herbalist is that they allow us to buy the plant by weight.

Aside from these two conventional and safe channels to getting medicinal plants, there is yet another popular method that is much more difficult to control: the Internet. This large supermarket is an attractive showcase for all kinds of products, and plants are no exception. But just as you would do purchasing food, drugs, and so forth, go warily on the Web. Even more so, considering that, according to recent data published by the Ministry of Health, 10 percent of the medicines sold online are fake. As for the plants, there are many websites where you can find all kinds of herbal remedies; the problem is that many of them lack proper sale warranties, and some sellers distort or exaggerate their medicinal properties and effects for purely commercial purposes. So the authorities have sounded the warning bell for greater control of these types of businesses.

Drugs or traditional medicine?

Today there is a clear distinction between medicinal plants that are considered medications and approved by health authorities that can diagnose, prevent, or cure diseases and those herbal medicines with more traditional uses. The first are plants that are sold with directions (which have been authorized by the Ministry of Health and supervised by the Medicines Agency) and can only be purchased at pharmacies. The latter are medicinal plants that are used traditionally and sold freely without reference to their therapeutic, diagnostic, or preventive properties. These are exclusively ingested, inhaled, or applied topically; they are mostly harmless, and their usage is based on people's experience with them over the years.

In general, despite the fact that herbal medicine is increasingly accepted and that the World Health Organization (WHO) recognizes their unquestionable capacity for treating a wide range of health problems worldwide, there is no legislation regulating phytotherapy, which would allow mentioning the health effects of medicinal plant based products. In Spain, the Law of Medicine is responsible for regulating products made from medicinal plants only through Article 42: "Plants traditionally regarded as medicinal may be freely sold to the public as long as they are offered without reference to therapeutic, diagnostic, or preventive properties; their sale by street vendors is prohibited." This means that outside of the pharmaceutical industry, the law prohibits labeling containers with medicinal properties of a plant, so that it cannot be marketed as a drug.

This same law states that "The Ministry of Health will establish a list of plants whose sale to the public is restricted or prohibited because of their toxicity." Currently the list numbers 197, although in some cases not the whole plant is prohibited, just some of its parts. Their use is restricted to pharmaceutical fabrication, homeopathic treatment, or laboratory experiments. Among these, there is coltsfoot (*Tussilago farfara*), whose whole plant is prohibited; com-

What you need to consider

- When plants are packaged in products, be sure to check that they include dosage information, lot number, and expiration date.
- If you are not used to taking herbal remedies, it is best to start with tablets and capsules that are made using the whole herb or dry powdered extract and that have highly concentrated active ingredients.

- If you want to try using a mixture of different plants or some magic formula, it is best to let the herbalist put it together for you, so as to ensure proper dosage for it to be effective.
- The same applies for tinctures. Although you can purchase them pre-prepared, it is best to order them from an herbalist or pharmacy in an amount that meets your therapeutic needs.

frey (*Symphytum officinale*), which is also prohibited in whole; and mistletoe (*Viscum album*), whose fruit and leaves are prohibited.

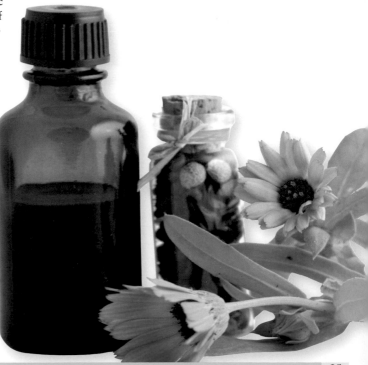

Endangered plants

The gain in popularity of herbal medicine has contributed to the overexploitation of certain plants. Unsustainable agricultural and forestry practices and the accelerated pace of environmental destruction have led to a situation that threatens the conservation of more than 10,000 species from among the 50,000 to 70,000 plants that are known for their medicinal properties. Some of those at risk of disappearing are grown in poor countries, such as the Amazonian rainforests or in the Andean region, and many others grow in the wild (they are much more vulnerable).

At the moment, more and more institutions, organizations, and working groups involved with the conservation of medicinal plants and nature in general are launching a series of initiatives and strategies to prevent the disappearance of these species, regionally and internationally. A significant example is the publication of the World Conservation Guidelines of Medicinal Plants, carried out by different international organizations, led by the World Health Organization and the World Wide Fund for Nature. They provide a set of guidelines on good agricultural and harvesting practices for medicinal and aromatic plants, as well as standard operating procedures. They also promote sustainable farming and harvesting methods that encourage the conservation of these species and the environment in general.

It concerns us all to get this situation under control. Beyond being a valuable therapeutic resource, medicinal plants are an important component of the planet's biodiversity. As consumers, you can help by taking a simple first step: buy only those species that have been produced and harvested in a sustainable and ethical manner.

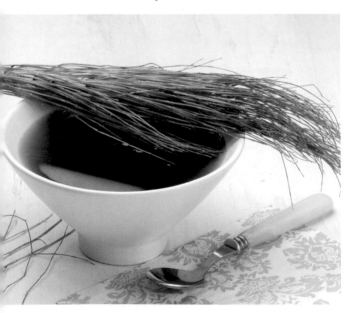

Buy with Your Head

When purchasing medicinal plants to make your remedies, it is important to do so in establishments that guarantee that their products are produced and harvested in an ethical and sustainable manner.

Some examples

- Ginseng (*Panax ginseng*)
- Horsetail (*Equisetum arvense*)
- Boldo (*Peumus boldus*)
- Arnica (*Arnica montana*)
- Ipecacuanha (*Psychotria ipecacuanha*)
- Quina (*Cinchona succirubra*)
- White nettle (*Lamium album*)

Chinese herbal medicine

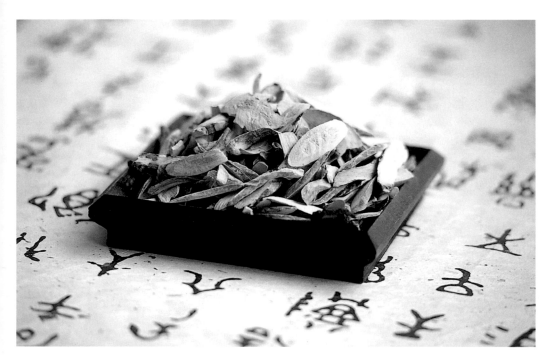

Traditional Chinese Medicine (TCM) is an ancient science; although it became known in the West in the thirties, it is more than four thousand years old. According to relics and historical documents, acupuncture dates back to the Neolithic period, and the oldest writing on TCM dates back to the eleventh century BC. Since the seventies, the World Health Organization began to pay attention to China's success in solving their health problems, so that in 1975 it created the Promotion and Development of Traditional Medicines program. Today, as TCM is becoming better known in the West, scientists and doctors from Chinese hospitals and universities conduct rigorous scientific studies on the efficacy and safety of different therapeutic treatments (herbal medicine, acupuncture, moxibustion, etc.), which contribute greatly to their development and dissemination worldwide. More and more people are using TCM to treat their health problems when Western orthodox medicine does not cure them.

A wise choice

Among the thousands of existing plants, TCM doctors use about 300 species, not only to cure certain ailments but as preventive medicine designed to strengthen and tone the body.

Basics of Traditional Chinese Medicine

TCM takes a holistic approach that is based on the idea that you cannot understand the parts outside of their relation to the whole; that is, if a person has a symptom, TCM aims to figure out how that symptom fits into the patient's overall condition. Its therapeutic system is extremely well developed and refined, and it rests on four pillars: herbal medicine, acupuncture and moxibustion (applying heat to the skin surface), tuina (massage techniques), and Chinese diet.

Using plants

Undoubtedly, Chinese herbal medicine is the most widely accepted unconventional therapy system with the greatest dissemination throughout the West. The repertoire of traditional Chinese remedies is one of the most comprehensive sources (contains more than 7,000 species of medicinal plants) and best documented that exist. It has been continuously used throughout history. It is interesting to note that it includes vegetables, mineral substances, and animal species. There are many remedies that are used in Chinese herbal medicine. The following are a few examples that have recognized therapeutic value.

Goat's thorn
(Astragalus gummifera or membranaceus)

Although it is native to China, it is now distributed worldwide. In Chinese herbal medicine, goat's thorn is usually mixed with other herbs, and it has been used for thousands of years to treat general weakness and chronic illnesses and to increase vitality. No wonder it is considered one of the most important tonic adaptogens. Now it is also used to treat heart disease, liver disease, kidney disease, cancers, viral infections, and immunodeficiency.

In the West, some studies have demonstrated its ability to stimulate the immune system with potent antiviral activity. Its potential use for treating immune deficiency diseases is also being studied, as adjunctive therapy against cancer (especially of the liver) and for its adaptogenic effect on heart and kidney disease.

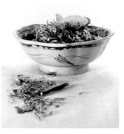

Shiitake
(Lentinus edodes)

Shiitake is a fungus native to eastern Asia that was not in our flora, but now, thanks to modern technology, it is grown in greenhouses in many countries. It is sold fresh or dried, is very aromatic, and has a great taste, so in addition to its medicinal properties, it is prized for its culinary uses.

In Japan, China, and Korea it has been known and used for centuries mainly for its tonic-energetic effect. In the West, it has been widely studied for the past several years, and, for now, it has demonstrated an ability to stimulate the body's defenses. It is used as adjunctive therapy to boost the immune system for patients undergoing chemotherapy and radiotherapy treatment. It has also been included in several experimental compounds in the fight against AIDS. It is currently being tested for possible antiallergenic, anticancerous, and antiviral effects.

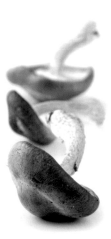

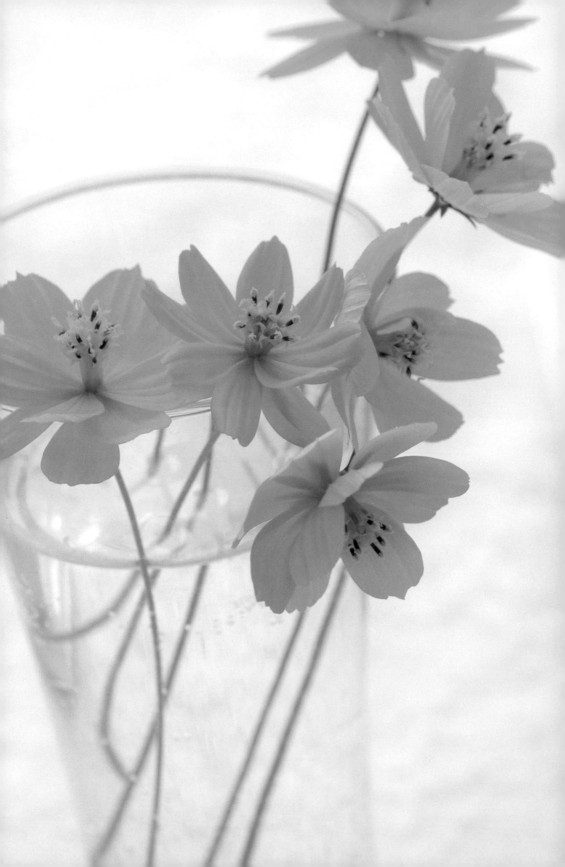

For all

Medicinal plants

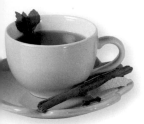

For the traveler

To avoid turning a day trip into a day of bed rest, the best solution is to have a well-stocked first-aid kit. For minor ailments, plant-based remedies can restore your health quicker than certain synthetic drugs. Although herbal teas are very effective, and they offer great healing properties, they may be impractical to prepare because you may not have a source of drinking water nearby or the right tools. For this reason, herbal capsules and tablets or tinctures are more convenient. In the following pages, you will find some common health problems you could encounter while traveling and ways you can fix them quickly and effectively using medicinal plants.

For women

Hormonal changes in women are momentous, since they trigger different stages that women go through in life. The starting point occurs as puberty approaches, when the pituitary gland in the brain increases the secretion of follicle-stimulating hormone, which in turn stimulates production of estrogen by the ovaries. The resulting menstruation marks the reproductive years for women. This fertile period lasts from the first period (twelve to thirteen years of age) to the last (at around fifty). The lives of women are marked by changes that are directly affected by hormones. During these years, fluctuations in hormone levels may cause changes in women's health. Although in general they are unimportant disorders, there is a percentage of women for whom these disorders are so intense that they may require medical treatment. The most common are premenstrual syndrome, menstrual cramps, irregular menses, pregnancy-related problems—or other ailments that are not strictly related to hormonal imbalances, such as urinary tract infections or vaginal candidiasis, and which can be alleviated by using medicinal plants. The key is finding the most appropriate remedy in each case, following the expert advice of the herbalist, and getting the approval of the physician or gynecologist. Among them, soybeans stand as the best ally.

For pregnancy

During pregnancy, especially in the early months, many women suffer discomfort due to hormonal changes that occur at this stage. For pregnant women, some plants are safe and effective remedies while others that are useful and recommended in other stages of life can be dangerous for the mother and the fetus in the first nine months; that is why we have chosen those that can be taken safely.

For children

Instead of using drugs, which can be aggressive for children and have side effects, you can use certain medicinal plants to relieve common health problems. However, keep in mind that not all plants are harmless: elements of the plant, or the plant as a whole, could be contraindicated. Below, you will find a selection of safe herbal remedies for children.

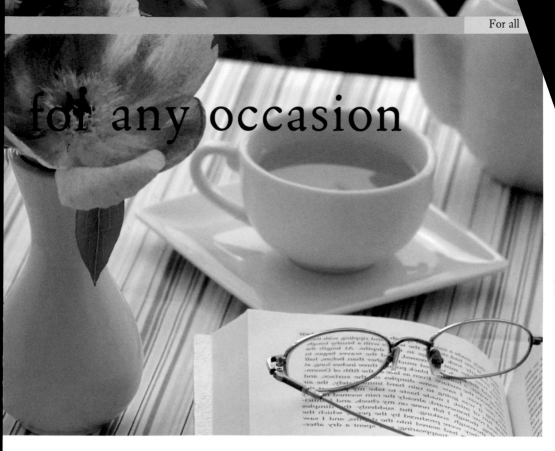

for any occasion

For men

Due to hormonal activity, women and men have different health problems. Men are at greater risk for cardiovascular disease, precisely because estrogen protects women during their childbearing years. After a certain age, it is very important for men to keep in check their cholesterol, triglyceride levels, and blood pressure. Other disorders that are specific to them are those related to the prostate. Just as women undergo gynecological examinations each year, men should do the same with the urologist to prevent further problems, especially starting at the age of fifty. Men can use medicinal plants to help them deal with sexual problems such as impotence or lack of desire, or other more aesthetic problems like baldness.

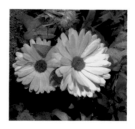

Antidiarrheal agrimony

(Agrimonia eupatoria)

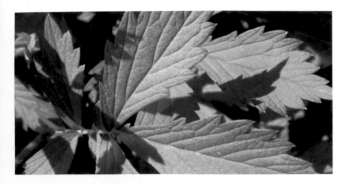

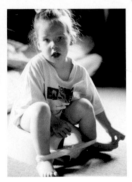

The most frequent health problem when traveling is called "traveler's diarrhea," which affects up to 80 percent of people who go to high-risk countries (Africa, Asia, and Central and South America) where the sanitary conditions of water purification, and food preparation and preservation, are not very safe. In many cases, it is limited to mild cases of diarrhea lasting two or three days, but it can make traveling difficult. In other cases, diarrhea is accompanied by fever, nausea, vomiting, and even dehydration. Diarrhea is mostly due to drinking polluted water and consuming food with toxins.

Why is it good?

For its tannin content, agrimony is considered an astringent that can be used to treat diarrhea.

Does it have other uses?

Precisely because of its richness in tannins it is also effective for gargling as a treatment for pharyngitis or tonsillitis. Using drops of agrimony helps treat conjunctivitis. Externally, it is an excellent remedy against dermatitis because it relieves intense itching.

How is it taken?

To stop persistent diarrhea, drink an infusion of agrimony that you prepare by mixing a teaspoon of the plant per cup of water. Boil it for two minutes, let it steep for fifteen minutes, and strain it. Drink three cups a day for three days to notice its effect.

Keep in mind . . .

- Do not drink tap water or use it even to brush your teeth.

- Do not eat raw fruits or vegetables unless they can be peeled and it is you who peels them.

- Do not drink bottled water unless the bottle is opened in front of you.

- Do not use ice made with tap water. If you do not know whether it was, drink your beverage without ice.

- Do not drink milk or dairy products that have not been pasteurized, that is, which have not been heated to kill all its germs.

- Do not eat undercooked meat or raw fish.

- Do not eat food sold in stalls.

Arnica for bruises

(Arnica montana)

Bruises do not break the skin as wounds do, but they do damage underlying tissues. Bruising causes pain and swelling, and the affected area turns purple after a while. Bruises are not a big deal as long as the blow that causes them is not too violent. While traveling, especially with younger children, always expect there to be bumps or painful bruises. It is in these cases when you should use arnica, whose active ingredients provide instant relief.

Keep in mind . . .

- After getting hit or bumped, it is also important to apply cold compresses locally with cold water or ice.

- Do not apply ice directly on the skin, and do not use it for an extended amount of time to avoid frostbite.

- Resting the injured area is important as well as applying anti-inflammatory ointment or gel. Very severe or multiple bruises should be evaluated by a physician.

Why is it good?

For external use, arnica is recommended when there is local inflammation brought on by a concussion. It works by lessening the bruises and blood clots that accumulate under the skin.

It should be applied to the injured area as soon as possible, in diluted doses for people with sensitive skin, as it can be irritating and cause allergic reactions. It should never be applied to open wounds. If used for a prolonged period, it can cause swelling and sores on the skin.

Does it have other uses?

Besides being an effective treatment for shock, arnica alleviates muscle tears and frostbite, as well as inflammations caused by rheumatism. It is recommended for external use only.

How is it used?

Arnica is available as a powder, tincture, and oil, which are used to prepare ointments, plasters, or creams, and then applied to the affected area three times a day. It can also be found in liquid extract and as dry and crushed plant ready for making infusions. In fact, you can prepare an effective remedy with a few tablespoons of fresh or dried arnica macerated in olive oil for two or three weeks. Then, with a bag of gelatin, filter it and keep it in a clear glass container. Use it to massage the affected area two or three times a day for reducing pain and swelling.

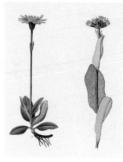

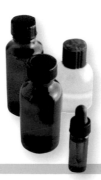

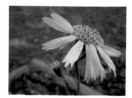

Marigold to treat bites & stings

(Calendula officinalis)

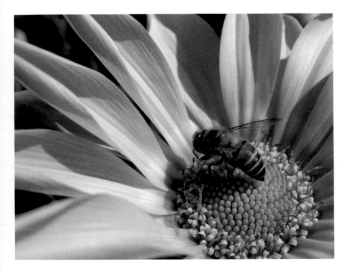

Why is it good?

Externally, marigold has potent anti-inflammatory, antiseptic, antibiotic, and healing properties. As such, it is an effective herbal remedy for protecting the skin to treat insect bites and stings, neutralizing the progression of the infection, reducing the resulting inflammation, and relieving any symptoms.

Does it have other uses?

This plant with beautiful yellow flowers is actually one of the most useful remedies provided by nature to cure a variety of skin conditions. It is also recommended for mild sunburn, scalding in the kitchen, bruises, bumps, and for treating eczema, boils, and pimples. It accelerates wound healing and stimulates cell regeneration.

How is it used?

Its flower heads (mixed with lavender, if you like) are macerated into compresses and placed on the affected area. Its tincture is diluted in water and used for massage. Marigold oil can also be used as the main ingredient in lotions, creams, or ointments.

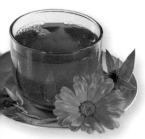

In summertime, the most frequent offenses are those of wasps and bees, who sting with a weak poison. A few stings are not harmful and only cause swelling and severe local pain. Although mosquito bites are not as painful, they tend to cause a lot of itching and are very annoying. As such, they are more of a concern for those who spend their vacations outdoors, so it is important to know how to treat them.

Keep in mind . . .

After an insect bite or sting, the skin becomes inflamed and irritated, so wash the area in cold water with mild soap, and then apply a natural treatment to reduce the swelling and burning sensation.

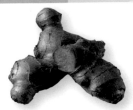

Ginger for dizziness

(Zingiber officinale)

Dizziness is characterized by a sense of instability. There are basically two types of dizziness: one is brought on by physical ailments, and the other is caused by motion (travel, sudden movements, certain types of entertainment, etc.). For this last kind of dizziness, ginger is a good ally.

Why is it good?

Among its many virtues, herbalists recommend ginger as a natural solution against motion sickness, dizziness, and feelings of imbalance. It is also recommended for morning sickness.

Does it have other uses?

Ginger stimulates digestion, increases salivation, and prepares the body to receive food. It stimulates appetite, especially after recovering from a disease or gastrointestinal illness. It relieves gastrointestinal spasms, and prevents gas and flatulence, which are also very common during pregnancy. Moreover, it is recommended as a treatment for respiratory conditions such as influenza, bronchitis, and pharyngitis.

How is it taken?

To relieve dizziness, especially while traveling, the best thing to do is to take one or two ginger capsules every four hours, starting half an hour before embarking on a journey and continuing throughout. If you forget to take ginger in advance, take it as soon as you start noticing any symptoms. If you are able to prepare a tea, boil a cup of water and remove from heat. Then add to it two teaspoons of powdered or grated ginger root, let it steep for ten minutes, and filter it.

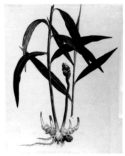

Keep in mind . . .

To reduce the risk of motion sickness it helps to do the following:

- Look out the front windshield, not through the side window of the car.

- Stay busy singing, talking—but above all, avoid reading while the vehicle is in motion.

- Make sure that air is flowing throughout the car, and no one should smoke inside it for the duration of the drive. The ideal temperature is 68° to 72° F (20° to 22° C), and it is recommended that you place shades on the windows.

- Make a rest stop every two hours.

- Avoid overloading your stomach before leaving. It is better if you eat dry foods rich in carbohydrates and avoid soft drinks and milk. During the trip, you can eat some cookies, chew gum, or eat candy.

- In a boat, try to stay as close to its center of gravity; avoid the deck because looking at ocean waves may cause motion sickness.

- On a plane, it is better to travel in the seats closest to the wings, where movement is less noticeable.

- As a preventive measure, instead of taking pills or gum to prevent seasickness, drink chamomile tea (two cups a day after meals).

Disinfecting **lemon**

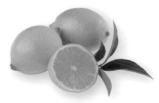

(Citrus limonum)

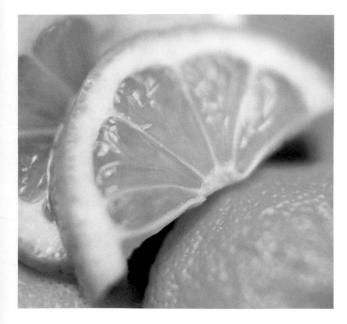

How is it used?

To disinfect and heal a wound, nothing beats lemon. For a major injury, the main thing is to stop any bleeding, so cover the affected area with sterile gauze and press with your hand to make it stop. For a sore throat, on multiple days gargle with the juice of a quarter of a lemon dissolved in half a glass of warm water. Another effective remedy is to drink lemon juice dissolved in water together with a clove of crushed garlic, for its antibiotic properties. Another soothing drink is made by mixing lemon juice with a little honey and warm water.

If bruises are common while traveling, injuries are no less common: slipping, falling, getting scratched. For these cases, there are natural solutions.

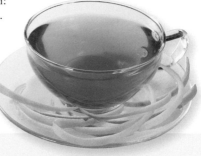

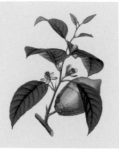

Keep in mind . . .

Clean the wound with soap and water. Then apply antiseptic iodine solution and place sterile gauze over it. Note: wounds have to be allowed to heal, no matter how small they may be. Also, if you are not vaccinated or did not get booster shots, you should see a doctor to seek vaccination against tetanus.

Other plants that are beneficial
for travelers

Siberian ginseng

Siberian ginseng is the best remedy to avoid confusion after a long flight. Take ginseng tincture or ginseng dried root capsules (a few drops or two capsules three times a day, beginning one or two days before the flight and ending upon reaching your destination).

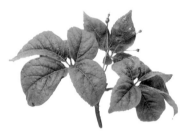

Saint John's wort oil

It is a good remedy for cuts and scratches. If you want to prepare it at home, place bits of the plant inside a glass jar and fill it with oil. Cover it and place it in a sunny location (like a window), and let it steep for two to six weeks. Filter this mixture, then store it in a dark glass container with hermetic seal. To use it, you only need to apply it on the affected area two or three times a day.

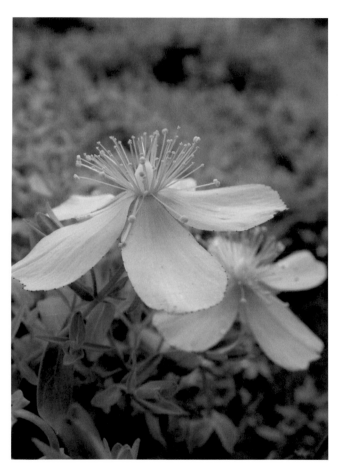

More remedies for your travel kit

– Matricaria capsules for headache
– Echinacea tincture for colds and flu
– Valerian tincture or tablets for insomnia
– Witch-hazel eye drops for mild conjunctivitis
  – Garlic capsules for infections

Ginkgo for your memory

(Ginkgo biloba)

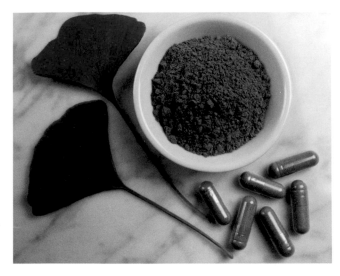

E xercising the mind is a good way to keep it healthy for longer, and it also helps to keep your memory and concentration in good condition. Regardless of your age, there is always time to activate your memory. The important thing is to stay curious, because being interested in everything around us lets our brain absorb and retain information. Reading, writing, board games, and conversation are ideal for exercising particular areas of the brain associated with language, numbers, reasoning, and spatial organization. In addition, some plants can be very helpful.

Why is it good?

Ginkgo works on the entire circulatory system, improving blood circulation, capillary circulation, and venous circulation. It is precisely this ability to improve blood flow that makes it an effective remedy to strengthen memory and delay aging.

Does it have other uses?

It protects the capillary, and has vasodilatory and venotonic properties, making it a very suitable remedy against cerebral circulatory shock, varicose veins, phlebitis, tired legs, and swollen ankles.

How is it taken?

It is best used in dosed capsules, tablets, and liquid extract. Although the dosage is already recommended in these products, it is best to consult with a physician. In pharmacies, you can buy medicines made with ginkgo, but always with a prescription.

Keep in mind . . .

- The importance of reading: it is a good way of exercising the mind; it helps to focus our attention and retain more information. Try to remember what you read.

- Crossword puzzles are a good exercise that forces us to think, use our memory, and satisfy our curiosity for new knowledge.

- Imagine and write: to jog your memory, you can start by describing what happened to you during the day. Try coming up with a story to strengthen your imagination.

Alfalfa for your bones

(Medicago sativa)

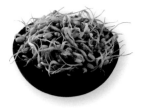

Bones are definitely weaker in older adults. Aging is the inevitable factor that causes their wear and weakness. From the ages of twenty to forty, bone mass is formed at the same time as it decays and maintains its density. Subsequently, especially in women after menopause, bone density and strength tend to decrease. This explains the higher incidence of osteoporosis and other bone diseases in women. Women have less bone mass development in comparison to men, and in Spain just as in many other countries, women tend to live longer.

Why is it good?

Much like soybeans, alfalfa is rich in vitamins and minerals as well as isoflavones. It has a detoxifying effect, it is rich in vitamins, it is restorative, and it has anti-anemic properties and estrogen. Compared to soybeans, its ability to prevent the onset of osteoporosis in postmenopausal women is much less known. It contributes to the strengthening and calcification of the bones, helps strengthen bones damaged by fractures, and prevents fractures when there is a propensity to develop osteoporosis.

Does it have other uses?

Alfalfa also helps to treat irregular menstruation and acts as a natural tonic for the anemic, weak, and convalescent.

How is it taken?

You can drink a simple infusion, two or three cups a day, or the juice of the fresh plant, or take it as a powder or in capsules. You can also consume it fresh in foods, salads, mixed vegetables, or sprouted seeds.

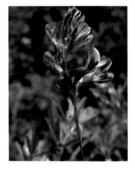

Keep in mind . . .

Aside from aging, there are other factors that damage the bones and should be taken into account:

- Incorrect diet: make sure you get an adequate intake of calcium (dairy products, broccoli, sesame seeds, almonds, sardines . . .) to help maintain bone health, and of vitamin D (cod liver oil, fatty fish, egg yolk, milk, and butter) for calcium absorption. Extreme thinness, especially after menopause, also weakens bones and affects proper nutrient absorption.
- Sedentary lifestyle: inactivity and lack of exercise work against bone health because they lead to poor muscle tone, stiff joints, obesity, and even osteoporosis.
- Stress: by increasing muscle tension, stress increases pressure between the bones, and it negatively affects calcium absorption.
- Some drugs: drugs such as cortisone, antacids, and anticonvulsants can be harmful to bones, mainly because some of their active ingredients block the absorption of certain minerals and vitamins essential for good bone health.

Garlic for your arteries

(Allium sativum)

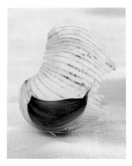

Cardiovascular health is crucial at every age, but over the years, the risk of certain diseases related to the arteries tends to increase because blood circulation becomes poor. During their reproductive years, women are protected by their hormones, but with the onset of menopause, this protection disappears. Smoking, a sedentary lifestyle, and a diet rich in saturated fat is harmful to the arteries. These poor habits form cholesterol deposits inside the blood vessel that get increasingly bigger and cause hardening and thickening of the arteries. If this process does not stop, it can clog and hinder blood circulation. Garlic is a good ally for older adults because it helps lower cholesterol, and it is a good blood thinner.

Why is it good?

The part of the garlic that you use is the bulb; commonly called a "head of garlic," it is made up of about ten to twelve "cloves." You could say that garlic is useful for practically

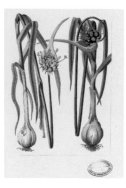

everything, as its properties are used for a wide range of conditions, mainly related to cardiovascular health. It reduces blood cholesterol levels, thins blood to prevent clots, and lowers blood pressure.

Does it have other uses?

Among other virtues, garlic has antioxidant, antiseptic, expectorant, and antimicrobial effects, and it boosts your defenses. In addition, it is an effective remedy to cure chronic bronchitis and colds. It is applied externally for treating calluses and warts.

How is it taken?

Garlic that you buy at any grocery store can be used for both culinary and medicinal purposes. Eaten raw, it is one of the best remedies that nature provides us to treat many ailments. You can also find garlic powder, capsules, as well as essential oil, all of which are practical options for those who want to avoid having garlic breath.

Keep in mind . . .

One of the biggest enemies of the arteries is high cholesterol. To prevent it, eat a balanced diet with plenty of fruits and vegetables, whole grains, fatty fish, white meat, skim milk, and olive oil. Do not eat saturated fats and sweets, and so forth. Practice moderate exercise, drink plenty of water, do not smoke, and avoid excessive amounts of alcohol (one glass of red wine a day at most).

Ash for osteoarthritis

(Fraxinus excelsior)

Osteoarthritis is a degenerative joint disease that alters articular cartilage and the underlying bone. It is the most common joint disease, and it mainly affects older adults. Although it occurs in both sexes equally, for women it is more common in the hand joints, while osteoarthritis in the backbone is more common in men. It should also be noted that some occupations in which the joints are used repetitively throughout the years predispose certain individuals to osteoarthritis (e.g., sewing, hairdressing, painting).

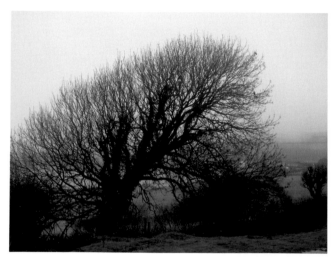

Why is it good?

Ash stands out for its diuretic and anti-inflammatory virtues. It promotes urination, and, in long-term treatments, it substantially reduces joint inflammation. It is recommended for reducing excessive uric acid levels and urea in the blood and as a treatment for rheumatic diseases such as osteoarthritis, arthritis, and gout. It is an excellent herbal supplement for people affected by periodic attacks of gout, to mitigate pain.

Does it have other uses?

Ash is a plant with diuretic properties, which makes it a good treatment against edema or fluid retention, as well as for relieving inflammation of the urinary tract, such as cystitis. Ash also has analgesic and venotonic properties, which is why it is recommended for varicose veins and hemorrhoids.

How is it taken?

Make a decoction (2 to 6 teaspoons per quart [10 to 30 grams per liter] of water), and drink three cups a day, preferably after meals. It is available as liquid extract (¼ teaspoon [0.5 to 1.5 milliliters] every 8 hours) and tinctures (½ teaspoon [2.5 to 5 milliliters] every 8 hours). It is also frequently used in capsules with powdered plant (the dose is indicated by the manufacturer).

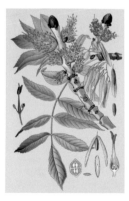

Keep in mind . . .

Although osteoarthritis is a degenerative disease, and, therefore, it is associated with age and repetitive joint movement, you should practice habits that promote bone health in general (see "Alfalfa for bones").

Bitter orange for your mood

(Citrus aurantium)

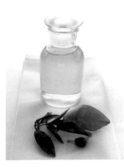

Nothing calms the mood of older adults more than the scent of bitter orange blossoms and leaves. They are especially helpful during stressful times, when they have trouble sleeping or staying asleep during the night, which is common for this age group.

Why is it good?

The essence of bitter orange blossom or neroli has the ability to ease nervous tension, especially when it affects the stomach. It is very effective for insomnia, nervousness, and palpitations.

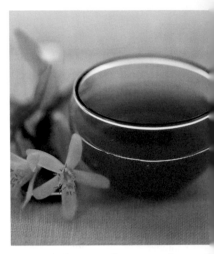

Does it have other uses?

Orange blossom infusion is also a very effective natural remedy for cramps, muscle pain, hiccups, bronchitis, and nervous cough. Orange rind, meanwhile, is used to tone up digestive functions and eliminate gas.

How is it used?

Given that its essential oil is the most active part of the plant, just take two to five drops (maximum) with a teaspoon of honey or a sugar cube or diluted in an infusion. You can also apply this oil to your daily bath or inhale it using a burner or a diffuser. It promotes relaxation and regulates sleep patterns. Another option is to add a few drops to vegetable oil (e.g., olive, almond), and use it to massage your chest, soles of your feet, and solar plexus.

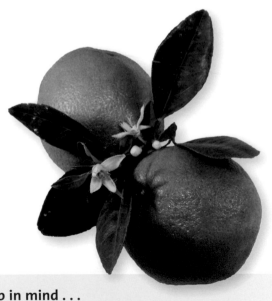

Keep in mind . . .

Doing moderate physical exercise and practicing relaxation techniques can help calm your tension and anxiety. Both yoga and tai-chi are recommended practices for the elderly because they do not require great physical effort, but they do work with breathing and mindfulness.

Other plants that are beneficial for older adults

Spirulina

As a dietary supplement for older adults, spirulina facilitates the absorption of nutrients (carbohydrates, fats, proteins) to transform them into energy. Spirulina is also used against anemia, by promoting red blood cell production. It is rich in chlorophyll, iron, and vitamin B12. Its omega-3 fatty acids help reduce cholesterol. It is sold as a powder that can be added to soups and salads (one tablespoon per person), and in tablets and capsules (follow manufacturer's instructions).

Fenugreek

This plant is recommended to combat listlessness that is common in older people. Its intensely colored seeds are high in protein (30 percent), flavonoids, saponins, and essential oil, which stimulate the appetite. It can be taken as a capsule or prepared as a decoction with a teaspoon of seeds per cup of water. Take ½ teaspoon (2 milliliters) of liquid extract with each meal.

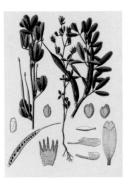

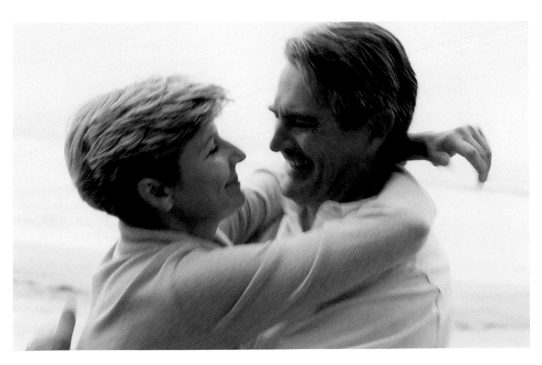

Soybeans, the great ally

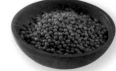

(Glycine max)

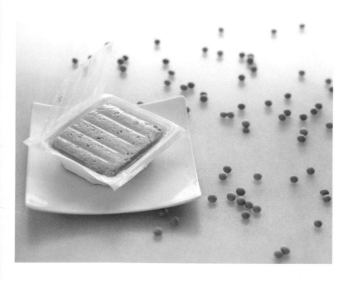

different studies have shown that in countries such as Japan, the risk of breast cancer is five to eight times lower than in Western European countries like Spain.

Why is it good?

Most of its health properties are attributed to isoflavones, being that they have a chemical structure that allows them to act in place of some female hormones, partially making up for estrogen, whose decline during menopause can cause hot flashes, irritability, insomnia, and ultimately, cardiovascular disease and osteoporosis. Specifically, eating soybeans reduces hot flashes by 30 to 50 percent.

How is it taken?

Each day, Asian women consume on average 40 milligrams of soy isoflavones, while the diet of Western women barely reaches 5 milligrams. To bridge this gap, experts recommend eating more food with phytoestrogens (legumes, especially soybeans, whole grains, and vegetables), or using pharmacological preparations. The active ingredients of soy have a half-life of eight hours in the body, so it is better to split the intake into two doses. Although you can eat it cooked, there are products you can easily include in your diet, for example, tofu, miso, tempeh, seitan, and shakes.

Undoubtedly, soy could be defined as an ally of women. It is very effective for preventing disorders associated with menopause that about three million Spanish women suffer—80 percent of them. It also works on cholesterol, helping to reduce cardiovascular disease, the leading cause of death in women over fifty. As if that were not enough, soy may also have a protective effect on bones. In this regard it is worth noting that the risk of osteoporosis is lower in Asian populations than in Western populations, and Japanese women have a lower risk of hipbone fracture than Western women, and this is directly associated to their soy consumption. Similarly, data from

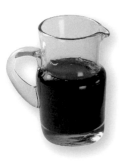

Chasteberry for menstruation

(Vitex agnus-castus)

Although the twenty-eight-day cycle is used as a standard, only 15 percent of the cycles of women of reproductive age last this long. Therefore, experts consider any period ranging from twenty-one to thirty-five days as normal. Each cycle is determined by bleeding duration, its intensity, and the interval between periods. Whenever there are fluctuations, we say there is irregularity. But do not worry, an isolated change is not a big deal; on the other hand, significant changes occurring over time should be discussed with your gynecologist, because in most cases they are due to hormonal problems that can be treated and cured. Besides inconvenient bleeding, such as that occurring outside the period itself, there are other bleeding disturbances affecting its duration or amount.

Why is it good?

Chasteberry is very effective as a hormone modulator to correct irregular menstrual periods, abundant and debilitating bleeding, painful periods, or when the period is excessively early or delayed. Chasteberry has an anti-estrogenic effect, and at the same time, it promotes progesterone activity from the pituitary gland. Herbal remedies made with this plant are especially useful for young women afflicted by irregular or painful periods.

Does it have other uses?

It is also recommended for PMS, breast tenderness, nervous irritability, and back pain, among others, as well as for relieving autonomic disorders associated with perimenopause. Moreover, its fruit has been used as a digestive stimulant, although its usefulness is very limited in this respect. Externally, the leaves are used as vulnerary (to heal sores and wounds).

How is it taken?

Prepare an infusion using only chasteberry, or in combination with other herbs such as sage, hawthorn, and viburnum (up to four cups a day). It is also available as capsules, tincture, and liquid extract.

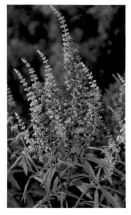

Keep in mind . . .

- Eat well: any eating disorder, a diet too rich in fats and proteins, strict diets, or eating disorders such as anorexia, can cause irregularities in the menstrual cycle or even loss of menstruation.

- Moderate exercise: strenuous or severe exercise can delay menstruation, since it can cause a sudden and rapid weight loss that affects menstruation.

- Stress free: it has been found that women who are subjected to high levels of stress, anxiety, and nervousness suffer from menstrual disorders such as irregular and delayed periods. It is therefore appropriate to try and lessen these stressful situations through relaxing baths or by practicing yoga.

Evening primrose for PMS

(Oenothera biennis)

A nother disorder related to menstruation is premenstrual syndrome (PMS), which is caused by ovulation. Its symptoms can include bloating, breast tenderness, fatigue, nausea, constipation, headache, skin disorders, irritability, anxiety, and sadness that do not disappear until menstruation begins. Its causes are not known, but PMS is related to hormonal changes (levels of estrogen and progesterone decrease in the premenstrual period) and psychological changes. Seventy-five percent of women suffer from it, although women who are in their thirties and have had children are more susceptible to it. It is also associated with stopping contraceptive use, or giving birth, and it is known that stress can make it more likely.

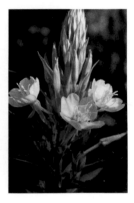

Why is it good?

To feel better in those days prior to menstruating, eat essential fatty acids (omega-3 and omega-6), which help with any symptoms. In this regard, evening primrose oil is a good source of fatty acids (especially gamma-linolenic acid), which increases the level of anti-inflammatory prostaglandins. It is ideal for relieving PMS symptoms such as bloating, discomfort, and painful breast tenderness.

Does it have other uses?

Among its many virtues, it is also used to prevent cardiovascular disease and relieve arthritis pain, and it is used externally against wrinkles, stretch marks, and pimples.

How is it taken?

The most common way of taking evening primrose oil is in liquid softgels containing a standardized dose, up to 1 teaspoon (6 grams) daily. Taken in low doses for ten days before menstruating, it substantially minimizes the symptoms of PMS. The oil can also be used in salad dressing, but that can be expensive. When used externally, it is an effective treatment for skin problems. For rheumatic pains, it can be applied by massaging gently.

Keep in mind . . .

- Diet: vegetable oils, oily fish, and nuts that are rich in healthy fats are also beneficial during menstruation. Eat foods low in salt, and drink plenty of water as part of your dietary habits to decrease fluid retention and other symptoms associated with PMS (e.g., bloating, constipation). Reduce your intake of sugar, caffeine, and alcohol. Increase your intake of complex carbohydrates and foods rich in magnesium, calcium, and B vitamins (especially whole grains, fruit, and vegetables).

- Relaxation: practice relaxation techniques to combat the physical and psychological symptoms associated with PMS by relieving muscle tightness, pain, and discomfort.

Black cohosh for menopause

(Cimicifuga racemosa)

Menopause does not just end menstruation, it sets off a series of major hormonal changes throughout the body, such as hot flashes, irritability, dry skin, and cystitis. The most important problems usually appear ten years later, and they are related to osteoporosis and cardiovascular disease. Although it usually occurs to women in their fifties, there are changes in menstrual cycle some months prior (e.g., amenorrhea, very heavy periods). This stage before menopause is known as perimeno-pause. The stage after the final menstrual cycle is called postmenopause, a period characterized by the changes resulting from the lack of estrogen.

Why is it good?

Black cohosh root contains an isofla-vone known as formononetin that, when released in the body, acts similarly to the female estrogen hormone. Several clinical studies have demonstrated its efficacy for treating neurovegetative symptoms associated with menopause, such as night sweats, frequent hot flashes, vaginal dryness, dry skin, headaches, back pain, dizziness, irritability, and insomnia.

Does it have other uses?

It is recommended for other gynecological disorders, such as dysmenorrhea, endometritis, or inflammation of the uterus and pelvis. However, it is contraindicated during pregnancy and lactation, as well as for those who have suffered from liver disorder.

How is it taken?

Black cohosh is taken in tincture, liquid extract, capsules, and more rarely as chopped or powder dried root. Make a decoction combined with other herbs such as sage and yarrow to reinforce its effect.

Keep in mind . . .

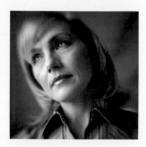

- Pay attention to your diet: after menopause, estrogen deficiency accelerates bone decay, which causes loss of bone tissue, also known as osteoporosis. The best prevention is a diet rich in calcium (found in milk, yogurt, and cheese) and vitamin D (such as in milk, fish, egg yolk), which enhances the absorption of the former. This vitamin is also obtained with moderate sun exposure. It is also important to exercise moderately, since lack of physical activity causes bones to lose mass and weaken. Note that excessive use of alcohol and stimulants such as caffeine and smoking also weaken bones and cause osteoporosis.

- Soy beans: in recent years, soy bean intake has been found to be beneficial in preventing symptoms of menopause. As stated above, recent studies confirm that Asian women who regularly eat soy usually have fewer problems than their Western counterparts.

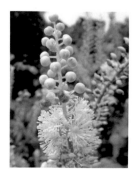

Blueberry to treat cystitis

(Vaccinium myrtillus)

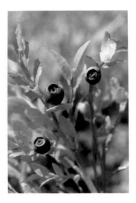

In addition to disorders related to hormonal changes, women are also prone to suffering urinary discomfort, such as cystitis, also known as urinary tract infection or bladder infection. It is estimated that between three and five out of every one hundred people suffer from it, mostly women, because the tube that connects the bladder to the outside (urethra) is shorter in women than in men. It usually occurs more frequently during pregnancy, when muscles of the urinary tract relax, and in general, in any situation that impedes urine from flowing easily (e.g., kidney stones), which allows bacteria to move up through the urethra and multiply. It should be remedied as soon as the first symptoms appear (e.g., pain or burning sensation when urinating and wanting to urinate even though the bladder is empty, hypersensitivity in the genital area) to prevent germs from spreading and affecting the kidney or other organs.

Keep in mind . . .

- Avoid tight clothing and fabrics that prevent perspiration, since moisture promotes bacterial growth. Your underwear should be made of cotton.

- Avoid harsh soaps, vaginal deodorants, and highly perfumed products, as these can irritate the vaginal area and destroy its natural defenses.

- Using spermicides and lubricants can cause irritation in susceptible women, and may lead to cystitis. Similarly, using a diaphragm is also a risk factor that increases the chances of cystitis. So keep the area well disinfected by using an antiseptic that your gynecologist recommends.

- Going to the bathroom frequently and completely emptying your bladder each time prevents bacteria from going up into the bladder, multiplying, and causing an infection.

- Drink plenty of water to prevent fluid retention, improve kidney function, and reduce the risk of infection.

- Eat foods like artichokes, onions, celery, and turnip (directly or as broth) to promote the production and elimination of urine and, therefore, lessen the risk of getting a bladder infection. Also reduce your alcohol intake, and eat fewer hot spices, fried foods, and pastries.

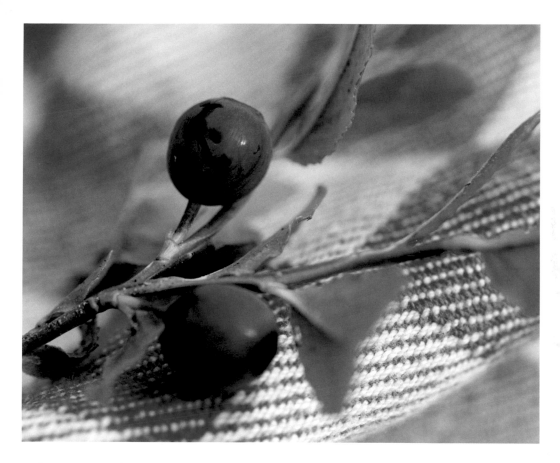

Why is it good?

Its leaves have a remarkable diuretic and antiseptic effect, much like many other plants in the heather family. Blueberries are effective at preventing and halting the spread of infection in the urinary tract, and are therefore a support for women affected by recurrent cystitis and other urinary tract infections.

Does it have other uses?

Blueberry leaves are also recommended as treatment for vaginal yeast infection, fluid retention or edema, and diarrhea. Externally, they can be applied to skin wounds and skin ulcers. Its fruits are rich in vitamin A and C, and mineral salts and sugars, so they are a good treatment for capillary fragility problems, such as varicose veins and hemorrhoids, and to treat vision loss and diabetic retinopathy.

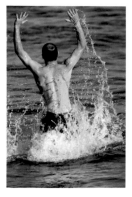

How is it taken?

Its fruits can be taken in capsules (with micronized powder), liquid extract, tincture (up to fifty drops a day, dissolved in water, three or four doses), or in fresh juice, and syrup. Use its leaves to make an infusion (one teaspoon per cup of water, three times a day).

Other plants that are beneficial for women

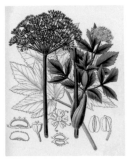

Angelica

Angelica helps with menstrual flow and provides vitality to counteract weakness caused by significant blood loss. It is a natural source of phytoestrogens, so it is ideal to compensate for the reduction in estrogen. It is taken in capsule or tincture.

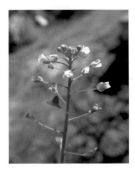

Sage

Massage sage essential oil on your belly (diluted in sweet almond oil) to relieve menstrual cramps. Use a clockwise motion covering the uterine and ovarian area. Massage daily for at least ten minutes so that the active ingredients of sage oil penetrate the skin. Its effect is noticeable after doing it for a month.

Clover

Clover is a good source of isoflavones, and recent studies have demonstrated its effectiveness as a hormone regulator, especially for reducing night sweats. It can help slow the loss of bone mass before and after menopause. It is usually taken in capsules or liquid extract, dry and crushed plant ready for tea, and as tincture.

Shepherd's purse

Shepherd's purse is recommended as an infusion or decoction (three cups a day between meals) for young women whose first menstruations are often irregular. It can also be taken in liquid extract and used as a compress.

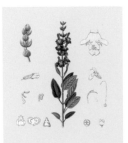

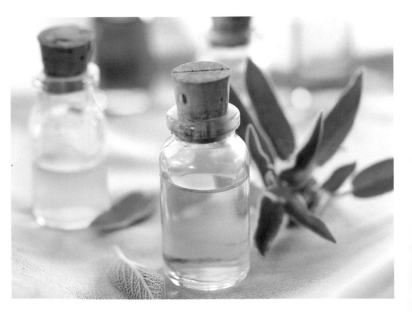

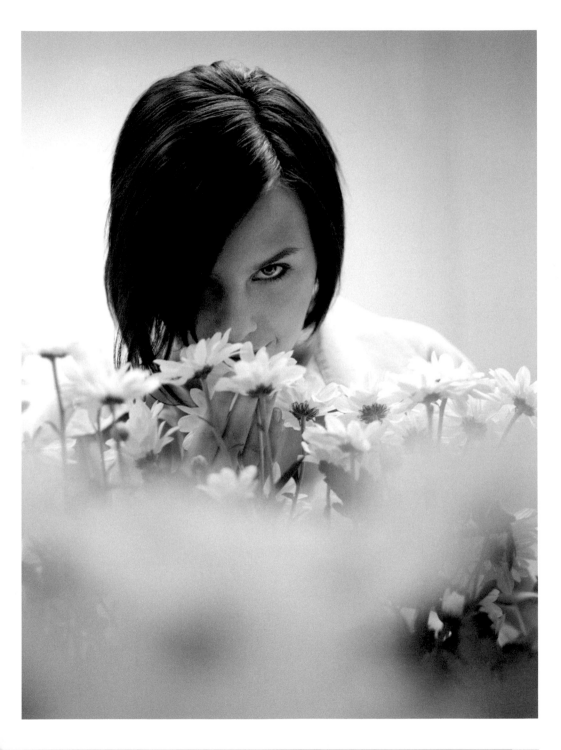

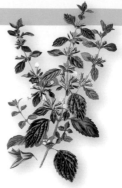

Lemon balm for nausea

(Melissa officinalis)

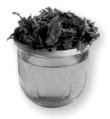

In the early months of pregnancy, it is not uncommon to feel dizzy, nauseated, and sick. To the dismay of many, the truth is that the exact cause of morning sickness is still unknown. It is likely due to hormone changes taking place during pregnancy and more precisely to hCG hormone (human chorionic gonadotropin) increase in maternal serum, which overstimulates the part of the brain that controls nausea and vomiting. Other causes may be gallbladder, hyperthyroidism, multiple pregnancy, and physical symptoms of pregnancy (intensification of the sense of smell, stretching of the uterine muscles, displacement of the digestive organs, and excess acid in the stomach). Stress and a high-fat diet may also be triggers.

Keep in mind . . .

- Eat small portions and do so often, every two or three hours, even if you are not hungry and before you notice any nausea. Dry crackers or toast are good snacks.

- Avoid foods high in fat content since they slow down bowel movement, which causes vomiting.

- Drink plenty of fluids, preferably ten to twelve glasses of water, fruit juice, or tea every day. Avoid alcohol and caffeine.

- Drink an infusion of fresh grated ginger (less than one teaspoon of powder per cup of water) in small amounts throughout the day to combat nausea and dizziness. Peppermint tea is also effective.

- Rest several times a day, lying with a pillow under your head and legs.

- If you are having morning sickness, eat a little as soon as you wake up, without getting out of bed. Ask your partner to make you something to eat or leave yourself a snack on the night stand. Do not get up right away.

- Move slowly and avoid sudden movements. After eating well, sit so that gravity helps keep food in your stomach.

- Avoid smells that make you feel disgust, dizziness, or wanting to vomit.

- Do not brush your teeth immediately after eating because that can cause vomiting.

- Try to get out and do some outdoor activities, like taking a short walk each day. If possible, sleep with the windows slightly open to let in fresh air.

Why is it good?

Lemon balm has a sedative action, which helps treat any nervous ailment (e.g., anxiety, nervousness, palpitations, insomnia, nervous headaches). It also works to treat dizziness, nausea, indigestion, heartburn, colic, flatulence, and other digestive disorders caused by stress.

Does it have other uses?

Its essential oil can be applied over herpes and wounds, and fresh juice of the plant is used to relieve stinging insect bites and minor wounds.

How is it taken?

During pregnancy, it is best to use dry and crushed plant in an infusion, and drink up to three cups a day. Do not ingest essential oil during pregnancy or lactation.

Sweet almond oil for stretch marks

(Prunus amygdalus var. dulcis)

Sweet almond oil is used to prevent and minimize stretch marks that usually appear during pregnancy especially on the breasts and the belly, because it stimulates tissue regeneration, and it provides active ingredients needed to repair the structures affected by traumatic stretching. By restoring elasticity, stretch marks are visibly reduced, and there is significant improvement in the texture and brightness of skin tone. Sweet almond oil is ideal for skin irritation and allergy problems.

Why is it good?

Originally from the mountains of Central Asia, almond has been cultivated since ancient times. It is well known for its beauty during its blooming period in late winter and for its nutritious almonds and valuable almond oil used for the care and beauty of the skin. Its oil is extracted by pressure from sweet almonds and has been used for millennia to improve the appearance and general condition of the skin, especially in cases of dry, dehydrated, or peeling skin. Today, it is widely used to manufacture lotions and cosmetics. It is very nutritious, especially rich in vitamin E, monounsaturated and polyunsaturated fatty acids, and minerals. It is suitable for all skin types, especially for the most sensitive, dry, or prematurely aged skin. It is used topically as an emollient, for its healing and anti-inflammatory properties. Aroma therapists and masseurs use it along with essential oils for therapeutic massages. It is their first choice because it is good for all skin types and is slightly relaxing. It is also used to give essences to children, older adults, and people who cannot tolerate alcohol solutions.

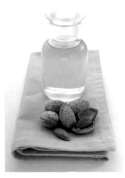

Does it have other uses?

Sweet almond oil, taken orally, has slight laxative properties. For constipation, the recommended dose is two to four tablespoons daily, preferably before breakfast. Sweet almonds, in addition to having excellent nutritional properties, help reduce cholesterol levels thus preventing cardiovascular disease, strengthen nerves, and tone muscles.

How is it used?

As treatment for stretch marks, apply almond oil twice a day on the affected area by massaging in a circular motion over the entire body. It can be used directly on dry skin, moist skin, after a shower, or added to bath water to enjoy a moisturizing, soothing, and very relaxing bath.

Keep in mind . . .

Use this oil or other anti-stretch mark product for massage to facilitate the penetration and diffusion of its active ingredients in an area where circulation is decreased due to breakage in the skin.
Avocado and avocado oil are also good for preventing stretch marks in pregnant women.

Corn, a major diuretic

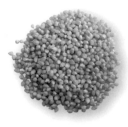

(Zea mays)

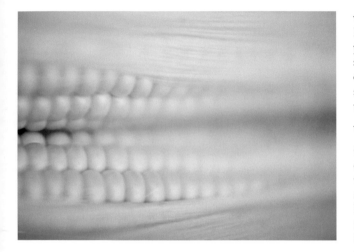

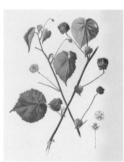

Through a complex system of hormones, our body is continually adjusting fluid levels to balance them, so that if you drink more water than necessary, nothing happens, because the excess is eliminated by the sweat glands or by the kidneys through urine. But when, for some reason, the body is unable to remove all excess liquid to maintain this balance, we have a fluid retention problem. Hormonal changes that occur during pregnancy often appear as a slight swelling of the ankles and feet. Mild edema can be easily treated, but you should never take any medication without consulting a specialist.

Why is it good?

Corn silk decoction is one of the most effective natural remedies to increase the removal of bodily fluids. It can also help with weight loss, reduce high blood pressure, prevent the formation of kidney stones or bladder inflammation, and prevent swelling associated with PMS.

Does it have other uses?

Cornmeal is applied externally in poultices for certain skin diseases, such as eczema, and to treat minor injuries. Corn oil is used in cosmetics.

How is it taken?

For internal use, make an infusion using its stigmas. It is also used as tincture, liquid extract, and capsules with dry extract. Moreover, corn oil is used in cosmetics for external use.

Keep in mind . . .

- Walk: moving your legs will help your kidneys work better.

- Drink plenty of water with low mineral content. The more water you drink, the more easily you will get rid of excess fluids.

- Get into water, whether in the pool, sea, or bath. Once inside, move your legs so that your muscles pump up liquid into your bladder. Water pressure will facilitate the expulsion of liquid through urine.

Restorative **brewer's yeast**

During pregnancy and lactation, the body needs an increase of B vitamins (especially folic acid), as well as magnesium, calcium, and iron. Take a dietary supplement that complements your natural food intake to meet nutritional needs.

Why is it good?

Brewer's yeast is the best natural source of vitamin B complex. It is also rich in minerals (phosphorus, calcium, silicon, zinc, copper, iron), essential amino acids, and active substances. Its restorative and purifying effect improves skin, nails, and hair, and keeps them healthy and vigorous. It also contains active ingredients that work to boost your defenses and helps regulate intestinal function, renewing its flora. It is recommended for those suffering from vitamin B deficiency or mineral deficiency such as zinc or iron.

How is it taken?

Restorative brewer's yeast is taken in flakes, tablets, and liquid yeast (the

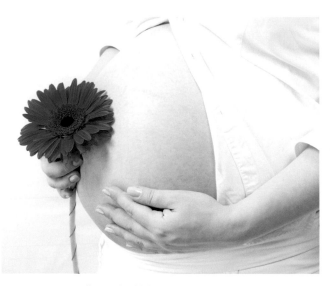

most nutritionally valuable). The recommended dose is 1 to 3 tablespoons (10 to 30 grams) per day. It can be mixed in soups, purees, juices, salads, yogurts, or cereals.

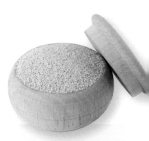

Keep in mind . . .

A balanced diet is essential during the gestational period, not only for the health of the mother but obviously also for the fetus. A healthy and complete diet helps prevent anemia and other deficiencies that may end up causing stress, fatigue, irritability, and other pregnancy symptoms.

Food must be whole and varied, and include vegetables, fruits, legumes, cereals (ideally whole grains), lean meats, fish, poultry, and preferably fat-free dairy products. It is important to limit your consumption of processed foods, pastries, sugary drinks, chips, and so forth,

since many of them provide a lot of calories and are of little nutritional value. Try to reduce your intake of animal fat such as butter, sausage, and pork.

Sand plantain
to prevent constipation

(Plantago psyllium)

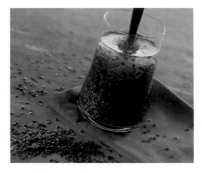

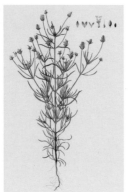

During pregnancy, many women suffer from constipation problems caused by an enlarged uterus compressing the colon, making fecal evacuation difficult. That is why constipation worsens toward the end. It is essential to drink plenty of fluids, eat foods rich in fiber, and walk every day. In addition, you can use sand plantain.

Why is it good?

Sand plantain's abundant mucilage explains its mild laxative effect, which does not irritate the intestinal mucosa. This is because when mucilage comes in contact with water, they swell considerably, and their volume increa-ses. Thus, fecal volume increases, stimulating intestinal peristalsis, and resulting in a healthy and effortless bowel movement. Additionally, mucilage drags out fats and other harmful substances, so that its laxative action also has a lipid-lowering and glucose-lowering effect.

Does it have other uses?

Sand plantain is anti-inflammatory and soothes mucous membranes, and it is also recommended for various gastrointestinal disorders such as heartburn, irritable bowel syndrome, and ulcerative colitis, and urinary diseases such as cystitis. Topically, this plant has been widely used to treat abscesses, boils, wounds, eczema, and burns. For all these external uses, it has been shown to have good anti-inflammatory and demulcent effects.

How is it taken?

Place a tablespoon of seeds in water and leave to macerate for half an hour. It should be ingested with another glass of water before breakfast, although it is best to take it already prepared, or in capsules or packets, without forgetting to drink plenty of water. If you feel abdominal pain for no apparent reason, do not take without first consulting a doctor.

Keep in mind . . .

- Fiber: ideally take about 6 teaspoons (30 grams) of fiber a day. To get as much, just follow a varied diet in which you include legumes, vegetables, and fruits.

- Drink plenty: fluid intake promotes intestinal movement.

- Exercise: lack of physical activity reduces bowel movement, which can lead to constipation.

Other plants that are beneficial for pregnancy

Aloe

This plant can be used during pregnancy without problems. It is ideal for skin care and burn treatment. Simply apply the aloe gel directly on the affected area.

Chamomile

This well-known plant has no contraindications during pregnancy, so it is good for treating indigestion and for aiding in relaxation before bedtime. Prepare an infusion with chamomile flowers.

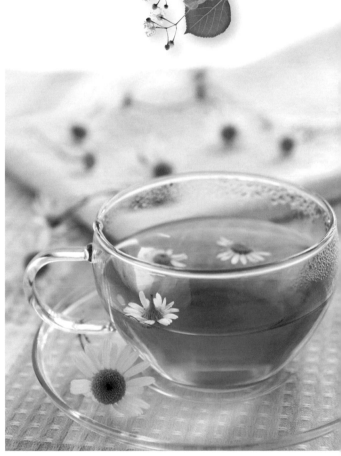

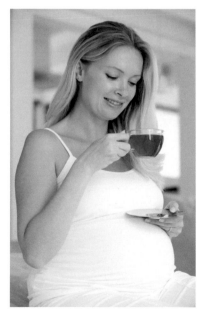

Avoid . . .

If in doubt, avoid consuming any herb during pregnancy. Likewise, avoid coffee since it can increase the risk of miscarriage. Do not drink alcohol since it gets through the placenta and can harm the fetus.

Chamomile for colic

(Matricaria chamomilla)

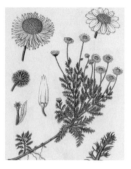

Colic is frequent in babies up to the age of four months: crying spells that last two or three hours and in which the baby is restless, has a red face, and stretches and kicks with his legs continuously. Although colic causes a lot of anxiety for parents, it does not mean that the baby is unhealthy, just that he is having trouble digesting food. To help the baby feel better, pick him up, rock him or rub his tummy using a circular motion. You can also try to calm the baby down by using chamomile, which is beneficial and harmless, even for children.

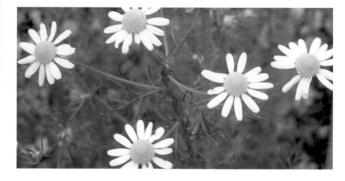

Why is it good?

Chamomile is a digestive and anti-inflammatory plant. It is considered an excellent remedy to relieve nervous indigestion, abdominal pain, and gastrointestinal spasms, and it is a good natural solution against colic. It also helps stop diarrhea, relieves general feeling of malaise and nausea, and prevents vomiting.

Does it have other uses?

As a sedative plant, it is recommended against nervous migraine, irritability, and sleeplessness, including insomnia in infants. Used externally, in bath water or applied as lotion, it alleviates skin irritations and rashes, eye inflammations, and rheum.

How is it taken?

For colic, even newborns can ingest it as a tea in very low doses, two small cups a day, after meals.

Keep in mind . . .

Besides using chamomile, if the baby suffers colic, pick him up so that his head is resting in the crook of your elbow and your hand reaches his diaper. The pressure of his stomach against your forearm will relieve the pain caused by intestinal gas. You can also massage his belly or do this exercise: with the baby on his back, bend his legs against his abdomen, gently, to help him relieve spasms and release gas.

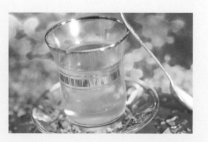

Hops for sleeping well

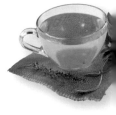

(Humulus lupulus)

Not all children need the same hours of sleep, but they all need a minimum amount to give them quality rest and allow them to carry out the day's activities normally without mood swings. Tiredness, headache, irritability, aggression, wanting to sleep at odd hours . . . these are signs that the child is not sleeping well. Some children will not need sleep nor show any symptoms despite sleeping little and not even needing a nap. Other children, even after getting enough sleep, may lack adequate sleep and not be well rested. Hops can help them get to sleep and ensure restful sleep.

Why is it good?

Hops belong to the Cannabinaceae family and, as such, is a powerful remedy that relaxes the nervous system. Therefore, hops are one of the best remedies for deep sleep and to reduce irritability and anxiety.

Does it have other uses?

This plant is also recommended against headaches and neuralgia. Furthermore, its sedative effect helps calm intestinal spasms. It is also considered a useful alternative to treat loss of appetite due to being upset or in a nervous state. In women, the soothing effect of the plant helps mitigate menstrual cramps, while its flowers help eliminate water retention.

How is it taken?

Hops can be taken in an infusion, which is prepared by mixing a teaspoon of cones (female flowers) per glass of water, without boiling, and letting it sit for ten minutes. Drink half a cup before bedtime. You can also place a small pouch filled with dried strobili in your pillow. Breathing the scent will help you get to sleep.

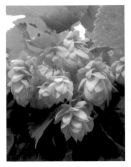

Keep in mind . . .

- The bed is only for sleeping: ensure that the child only uses it to sleep. Keep him from playing or watching TV in bed.

- Regular hours: babies are not the only ones who need a routine; children do too. So it is important to get up every day at the same time, no matter how much you slept at night. This will help you set a sleep pattern that is more restorative.

- Quiet room: the room that the child sleeps in should be isolated from noise, even if noise does not seem to affect him.

- Early dinner in an adequate amount: try not to let him go to bed on an empty stomach or, conversely, too full, because his sleep quality could be affected. It is also important to keep him away from drinks that contain caffeine in the hours before going to sleep (e.g., colas, coffee, tea).

- Do not force him to sleep if the child is not sleepy: the best thing to do when your child refuses to go to sleep is to get him to do a monotonous activity until he falls asleep (do not force him to sleep because that could cause him to establish a negative association with bedtime). But do not let him fool you.

- Regular exercise: make sure your child exercises regularly, as it will help him fall asleep more easily and stay asleep. Physical activity should be done in the afternoon and end well before going to sleep so as to avoid overexcitement.

Mallow for colds and flu

(Malva sylvestris)

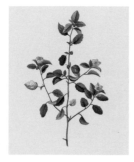

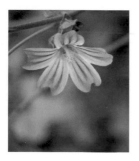

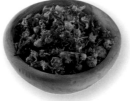

Several studies have found that catarrhal inflammation of the upper airways is the main reason that children in kindergarten and preschool get sick, and it has a higher incidence in children under two years old. Children also tend to catch the flu, and suffer gastrointestinal infections and certain skin conditions. Colds or runny noses are the most common inflammations of the mucous membranes in the fall and winter months. Its symptoms are well known: congestion, runny nose, sneezing, coughing, and sometimes a mild fever (99° to 100° F [37.5° to 38° C]). It is not a serious illness, but it can cause an acute otitis, especially in children between the ages of three and five, and sinusitis. The start of the school year often coincides with the dreaded flu virus season. It is similar to the common cold but includes symptoms of malaise and fever, headache, and joint pain. Today, we know that children are particularly affected and that they transmit it to adults.

Why is it good?

Mallow is a highly effective natural remedy to soothe sore throats or bronchi, reduce mucus, and relieve tonsillitis and all kinds of respiratory diseases as well as the flu.

Does it have other uses?

Mallow flowers are also used to regulate bowel movements because they are slightly laxative. Its infusion is an appropriate treatment for children and older adults who suffer from constipation. Externally, you can boil mallow flowers, drain them and apply them as a poultice to help eliminate pimples and boils on the skin.

How is it taken?

For cold or flu, syrup form is more effective. You can take up to three teaspoons per day. Infusion (three cups a day before breakfast) is better for treating constipation.

Keep in mind . . .

- Rest if you have a fever.

- Avoid smoking in front of children, as that may worsen their cold symptoms.

- Offer plenty of fluids such as water, fruit juices, and broths. Fluids help liquefy the mucus and eliminate it more easily.

- Eat foods that help you make a quick recovery: healthful fruits and vegetables provide vitamins, minerals, and antioxidants such as vitamin C, which boosts your defenses.

Horehound for cough

(Marrubium vulgare)

Cough is a common disorder in children and is one of the symptoms of colds that get transmitted between children in school. Indeed, fall and winter months are a critical period for health. Sudden changes in temperature and seasonal changes are primarily responsible for respiratory disorders, affecting people of all ages and sometimes turning into infections.

Why is it good?

The flowering tops with most of its active ingredients (especially marrubiin) are an effective remedy for respiratory conditions. Due to its expectorant properties, it is particularly suitable for treating colds, bronchitis, acute asthma attacks, and all respiratory diseases accompanied by cough, because it makes bronchial secretions flow.

Does it have other uses?

It is a remarkable digestive plant that reinvigorates listless children, which is a common cold and flu symptom. Its syrup has a pleasant taste.

How is it used?

Horehound can be taken as a tea (two cups per day) prepared with 4 teaspoons (20 grams) of flowers per quart (liter) of water. However, for children it can be unpleasant because of its bitter taste. A good alternative is to add it to bath water. You only need 2 pounds (1 kilo) of flowering tops of horehound for 1.3 to 1.5 gallons (5 to 6 liters) of water. When it starts to boil, add it to the bath water. Bathe

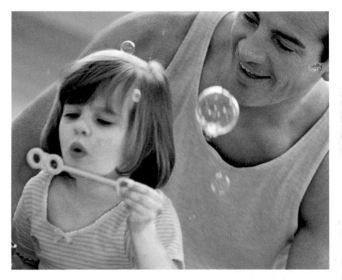

your child in this water, and repeat the process for two or three days until the cough begins to subside. You can also make syrup using fresh plant juice mixed with sugar or honey.

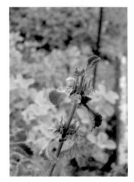

Keep in mind . . .

To soothe coughing, it is important to give children plenty to drink (water, juices, teas, soups). At night have them sleep with their head slightly elevated, and give them some propolis candy to soothe the throat.

Oats for dermatitis

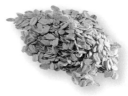

(Avena sativa)

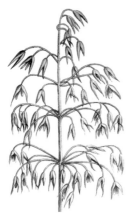

One of the most common skin diseases in children, from the time they are born, is dermatitis. Although there are different types, the most common is called atopic dermatitis, which affects 15 percent of children. Dryness and intense itching are the main symptoms that can appear in the first months of life. Symptoms usually improve by two or three years of age, and they become less severe as the child grows. It is unknown exactly what causes it, but it seems to be related to an immune disorder, and there is also a hereditary component. In addition, there are some factors that trigger skin inflammation: anything that dries out skin can aggravate atopic dermatitis, but it is especially triggered by soaps, detergents, perfumes, strong chemicals, as well as wool garments, temperature changes, hot baths, humidity, tobacco smoke, or dust mites.

Why is it good?

Oats, applied externally, are known for their dermatological properties. Oat extracts are used to make creams or oils for dry, sensitive, or irritated skin. They are emollient and regenerate and protect the skin from infections, providing smoothness and elasticity. These properties are attributed to their richness in polyunsaturated fatty acids, silicon, and mucilage.

Does it have other uses?

Oat straw and grains can also improve the mood of older adults and children. They are useful for treating depression, nervous weakness, exhaustion, and unwillingness to recover after a long convalescence.

Keep in mind . . .

Here are some tips to help you care for delicate skin of children:
- Clean their skin carefully so as not to disturb the skin's protective acid mantle against infections.

- You do not need to bathe children every day with soap, especially newborns, as this can alter the acidic lipid barrier and predispose them to dryness and infection. For this reason it is that you cleanse the newborn's skin and scalp only with warm water, and gradually incorporate scent-free mild soap.

- Room temperature should be neither too hot nor too cold; be mindful of any drafts and noise.

- Pay attention to the skin folds (behind the ears, neck, armpits, and groin area) and do not overlook the area surrounding the umbilical cord.

- Dry the skin using a towel or cotton cloth, without too much rubbing.

- Perfumes, colognes, and other scented products are not recommended as they may cause an allergic reaction.

How is it used?

For skin care, oats are used externally as oatmeal poultices, applied on the affected area. Oats are sometimes an ingredient in bath gel and body cream to improve dry and delicate skin. You can also use oat flakes and bran to prepare decoctions (2 tablespoons of oat grains per 4 cups (1 liter) of water). This decoction can be ingested and used in a bath to soften and hydrate the skin, as it eases away tension.

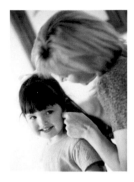

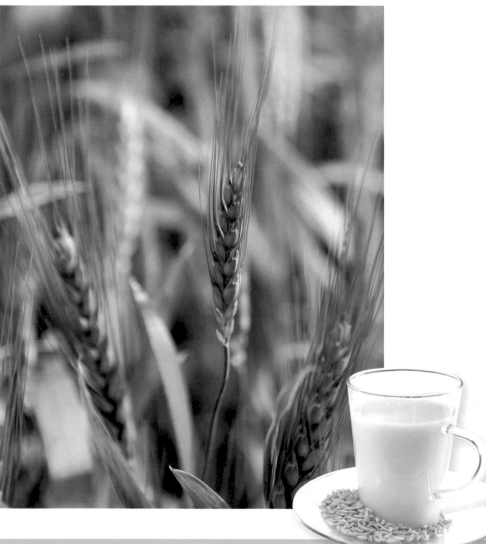

Other plants that are beneficial for children

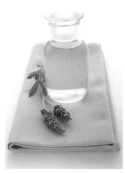

Lavender

Drinking two or three cups a day of infusion, or thirty drops of tincture, can be good for children three years and older so that they sleep more soundly without interruptions. Never give its essential oil to children.

Anise

Anise is another effective remedy for digestive problems in small children. It helps relieve gas, stimulates digestive functions, and eases fecal evacuation. Drink two cups of infusion daily; you can even put it in their bottle.

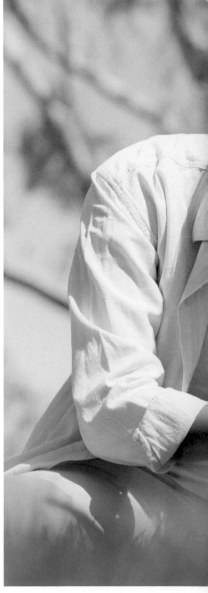

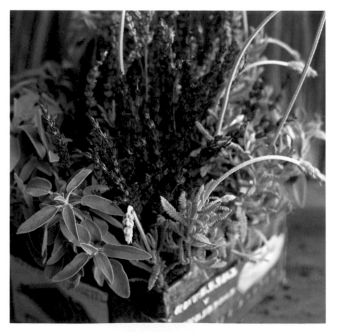

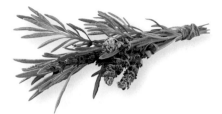

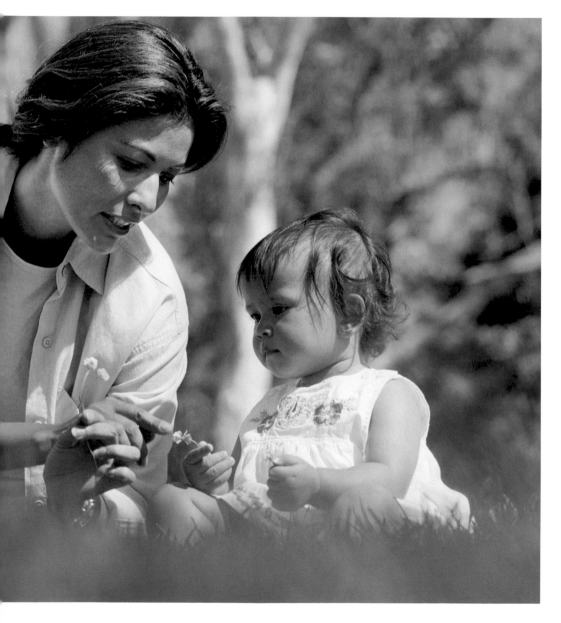

Saw palmetto for prostate

(Serenoa repens)

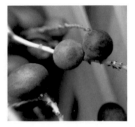

More than half of men over sixty have an enlarged prostate and risk having this gland grow over the years. As it enlarges, it gradually squeezes the urethra, making urination difficult and creating other urinary problems. In general, this growth is known as benign prostatic hypertrophy, and therefore it is not malignant. However, some symptoms may appear when the prostate gland has become so large that it interferes with urinary flow, such as feeling that the bladder is not completely empty, difficulty starting urination, or frequent urination. In some cases, prostatic obstruction can even cause repeated urinary tract infections, sudden inability to urinate (acute urinary retention), and increased kidney damage. This is where some plants, such as saw palmetto, can be useful.

Why is it good?

The dates of this small palm have been used for hundreds of years as a general tonic for the male reproductive system. According to recent studies, this berry or fruit is effective for prostate problems, such as inflammation or enlargement because it relieves congestion and inflammation, and it regenerates cellular tissue surrounding the prostate. Its benefits are attributed to fatty acids and sterols, active ingredients for maintaining the proper functioning of testosterone, the predominant hormone in the male reproductive system.

Does it have other uses?

It is also effective as a natural diuretic, purifier, and antiseptic, to treat urinary system disorders such as cystitis and kidney stones. It is a tonic that helps strengthen body tissues, so it has been traditionally used for testicular atrophy and premature ejaculation.

How is it taken?

Decoction (3 tablespoons of crushed dates per quart [liter] of water, boil for two minutes, cover it then let it steep for 10 minutes). Drink a glass before breakfast and another glass a half hour before each meal. Other intakes are liquid extract (15 to 20 drops in a little water, 2 to 3 times a day) and in capsules or tablets with dry extract.

Keep in mind . . .

Regardless of the prostate problem, follow these tips:

- Avoid obesity.
- Eat a healthy and balanced diet.
- Increase intake of fiber (e.g., fruits, vegetables, whole grains, legumes, dried fruits).
- Do not eat saturated fats (e.g., butter, meats, whole milk) or fast or frozen food.
- Reduce your intake of sugar and bleached flour.
- Reduce or avoid drinking alcohol and fizzy drinks.
- Avoid tobacco and other stimulants (coffee, tea, chocolate).
- Have a regular sleep schedule.
- Exercise moderately.

Buchu for urinary disorders

(Barosma betulin)

Urinary tract disorders are often associated with a blockage that prevents complete emptying of the bladder and often leads to urinary reflux. Urine accumulation in the bladder, ureters, or kidneys can cause infections and kidney failure over time. Some urinary tract disorders affect men because they are largely related to the male anatomy. From the southern tip of the African continent comes the buchu, one of the most popular herbal remedies in modern times for genitourinary problems.

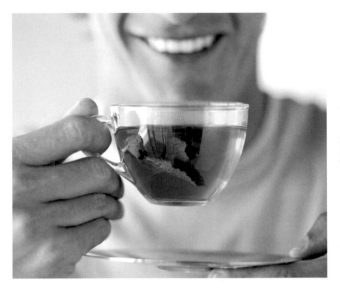

Why is it good?

The essential oil content of buchu's leaves is the main source of its antiseptic action on the urinary tract, making it very effective for treating acute cystitis and chronic urethritis. It is particularly suitable for those men who have difficulty urinating and who have prostate problems.

Does it have other uses?

Buchu is associated with all types of remedies that require an increase in urination, such as gout, edema, and high blood pressure. Buchu is also known for its purifying effect on the respiratory tract, so it can be used to treat colds, bronchitis, and pharyngitis. Its infusion can also be used as a tonic to eliminate stomach bloating and gas.

How is it taken?

Buchu is commonly used as an infusion (4 teaspoons [20 grams] per quart [liter] of water, in 3 doses per day). It can also be used as a tincture (up to 40 drops per day), syrup, and tablets.

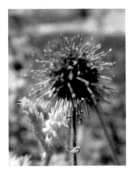

Keep in mind . . .

A healthy lifestyle is always recommended but more so to prevent such disorders: drink 8 cups (2 liters) of water a day; avoid alcohol, coffee, and stimulant drinks; eat plenty of fiber; and avoid saturated fat, salt, and sugar.

Damiana
for sexual disorders

(Turnera diffusa)

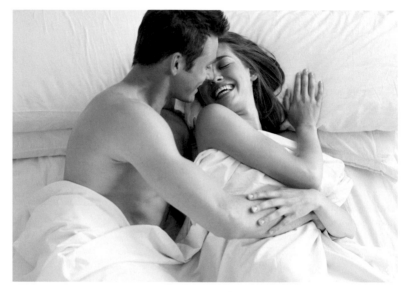

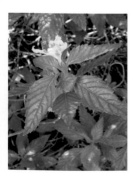

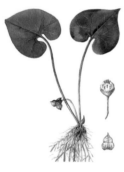

Impotence or erectile dysfunction, premature or delayed ejaculation, and low sex drive are some of the most common sexual disorders in men. They may be due to hormonal changes, disease, or medication, but often there is also a psychological component (anxiety, fear of rejection, or stress). While in some cases, sexual therapy is effective, you may also want to enlist nature's help by using plants such as damiana.

Why is it good?

This plant has a tonic and stimulating effect to restore sex drive, overcome premature ejaculation, and treat impotence. Its essential oil contains cyanogenic glycosides, simple phenols, and tannins.

Does it have other uses?

Damiana acts as an excellent nervous system stimulant, so it is recommended against mild depression and fatigue and puts you in a better mood.

How is it taken?

Drink it as an infusion (1 to 3 cups a day, not before bed), tincture (¼ to ½ teaspoon [2 to 3 milliliters] 3 times a day), or in capsules or tablets; the dose will be indicated by the manufacturer.

Olive for high blood pressure

(Oleo europea)

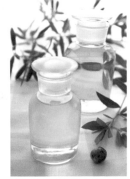

B lood pressure is the force exerted by circulating blood upon the artery walls of blood vessels. Generally, for an adult, normal blood pressure is between 140 mmHg and 90 mmHg. Hypertension occurs when blood pressure exceeds these numbers. The more difficult it is for blood to circulate through the arteries, the more the heart gets overworked, and the higher the blood pressure. Many people with hypertension do not know they have it because they experience no symptoms. So it is advisable to have your blood pressure checked regularly to make sure it is normal. This is especially recommended for men so as to avoid further complications; women of childbearing age are more protected from cardiovascular disease thanks to their hormones. Phytotherapy offers natural remedies to balance blood pressure.

Why is it good?

Olive leaves have a hypotensive action that dilates blood vessels and works as a diuretic, antipyretic, and antispasmodic. In addition, both the leaves and olive oil reduce high cholesterol levels. It is recommended for preventing coronary heart disease and other disorders associated with hypertension such as headache and vertigo. It is also used for treating mild circulatory disorders.

Does it have other uses?

Olives contain a lot of oil that is of great quality and takes a long time to become rancid, which makes it very useful to prepare numerous pharmaceutical medications. Specifically, it lowers cholesterol, it is slightly laxative, and, externally, it is an emollient.

How is it taken?

To take advantage of its hypotensive effect, drink three or more cups a day of an infusion made with a teaspoon of leaves (preferably fresh) per cup of hot water and letting it steep for ten minutes. The leaves can also be taken in capsule form, if you prefer. As for the oil, just take a couple of tablespoons throughout the day.

Keep in mind . . .

Besides using plants, it is important that do the following:
- Reduce salt intake.
- Follow a Mediterranean diet.
- Do not smoke.
- Avoid drinking excessive amounts of alcohol.
- Exercise.
- Keep stress at bay.

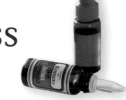

Rosemary for baldness

(Rosmarinus officinalis)

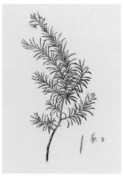

Hair loss affects men mainly due to genetic and hormonal factors (mainly by a hormone called dihydrotestosterone). It is called androgenic alopecia or common baldness. It occurs mainly in the forehead-temple area (receding hairline) and crown of the head. Psychosomatic factors such as depression and anxiety, infections, prolonged fevers, and unbalanced diet can also cause excessive hair loss by stopping essential nutrients from reaching the hair root. It is in these cases where plants such as rosemary can help, by revitalizing the scalp.

Why is it good?

Applied externally, its essential oil has a hypertensive effect (raises blood pressure) and invigorates the nervous and circulatory system. It also calms redness if you use it externally to stimulate the scalp. This same property is also used to treat rheumatism and lumbago.

The essential oil should not be used orally during pregnancy or lactation, for young children, or to treat gastritis, gastric ulcer, or epilepsy. Never exceed the recommended daily dose because it can cause irritation of the renal endothelium, and it is neurotoxic.

Does it have other uses?

Rosemary leaves have stimulant, antispasmodic, and slightly diuretic effect and are good cholagogues that promote bile secretion. They also have a tonic effect on the digestive system in general.

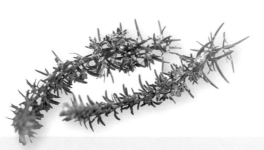

Keep in mind . . .

There is no doubt that stress and anxiety in modern life combined with dietary and environmental factors are contributing to baldness. Preventive and hygienic habits such as frequent, even daily, washing is advised as long as it is done using special shampoos. Do not use commercial products for hair loss unless they are recommended by a specialist. Protein and iron are an essential part of your diet (meat, fish, eggs, legumes, cereals, whole grains, etc.). You can also take a nutritional supplement (vitamin B6, B5 sulfur amino acids, antioxidants, etc.), as they are useful supplements that help and encourage the development of the follicle that may have stopped functioning.

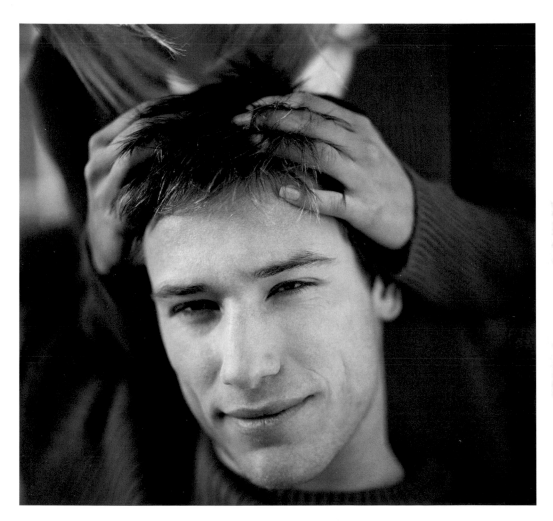

Infusion made with a teaspoon of rosemary leaves per cup of water promotes liver function, lessens intestinal spasms, and improves digestion. It is also good for nervous exhaustion and fatigue, as well as during a period of convalescence. It must be taken before or after meals. For external use, the decoction of rosemary applied to sores and wounds are an effective remedy because they have antiseptic properties.

How is it used?

If what you seek is to stimulate hair growth, the scalp can be rubbed with rosemary alcohol, which is made by dissolving 2 to 4 teaspoons (10 to 20 grams) of essential oil in 4 cups (1 liter) of 96 percent alcohol. You can also apply it to soothe rheumatic pains. If you prefer it, rosemary oil that is prepared by dissolving 4 teaspoons (20 grams) of essential oil in 4 cups (1 liter) of olive oil works very well.

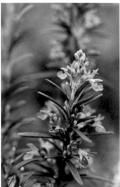

Other plants that are
beneficial for men

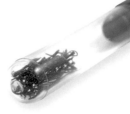

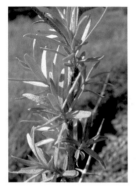

Hawthorn

Hawthorn is one of the allies of cardiovascular health and therefore is good for men. This is one of the best plants to strengthen the heart, tone blood supply to the coronary arteries, and prevent blood clots. Drink an infusion of the dried plant, at a rate of one or two cups a day. Yarrow and linden flower are also beneficial for hypertension. Mix them in equal portions, and make an infusion that you will drink warm, three times a day.

Saffron

Saffron is a spice with intense flavor and fragrant aroma that is widely used in cooking. It gives a characteristic orange color to foods. It is also known for its stimulating effects to counteract nervous exhaustion. It can be used as a condiment in your food, or as an infusion, sometimes mixed with cinnamon, up to .4 teaspoon (2 grams) per quart (liter) of water; drink 1 or 2 cups a day. It is also available as a tincture (up to 30 drops in fruit juice) and liquid extract.

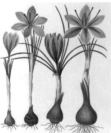

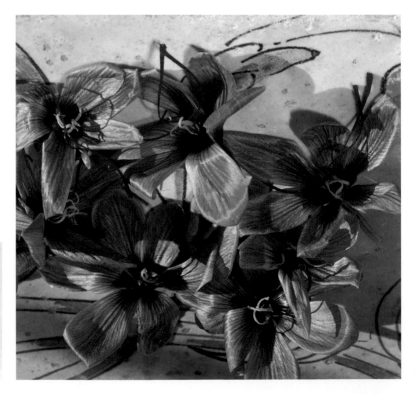

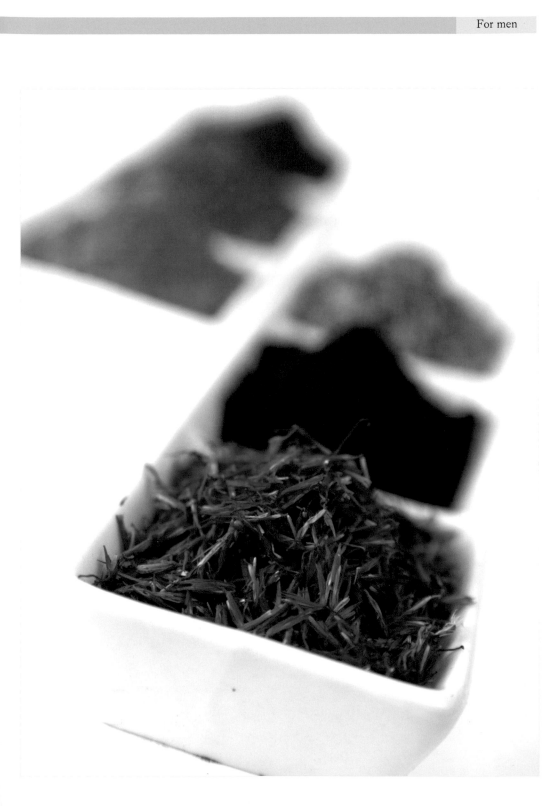

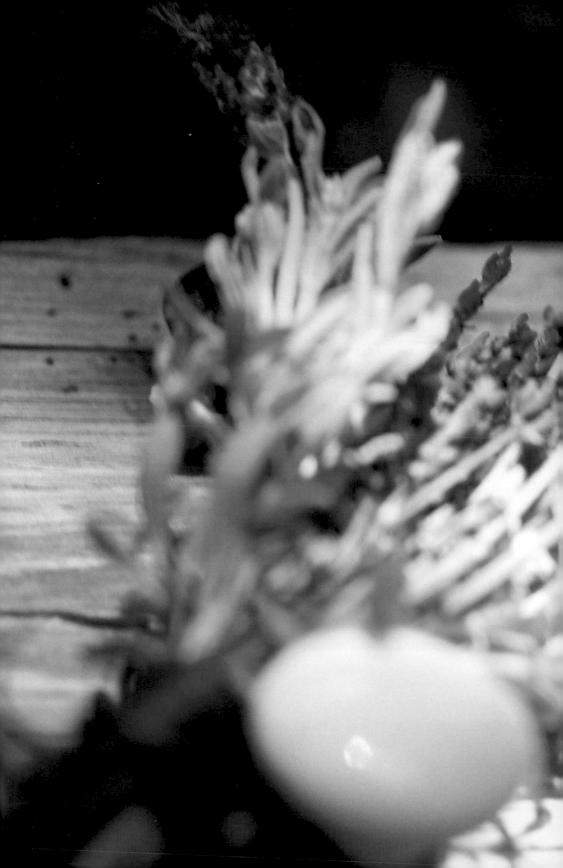

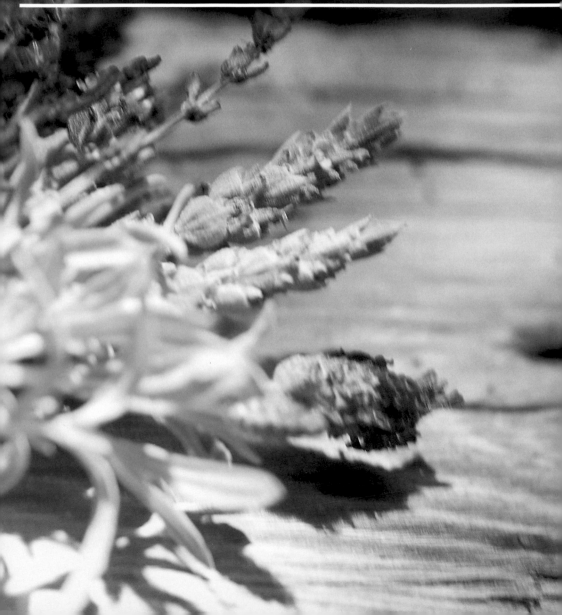

Throughout
the house

ON THE BALCONY

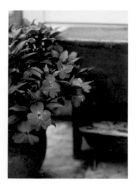

The benefits of plants are many, as you have seen so far and as you will see in the next chapter. You can get them at health food stores and pharmacies, or try to cultivate them for yourself. What? Many people hear the word "cultivate" and imagine a large orchard amidst nature. But it does not have to be that at all. Medicinal plants can be grown in a small urban garden or balcony. And you do not need to have a very large plot of land or invest much money. Water, light, and a good selection of plant species with beneficial properties for various ailments can make your backyard a true "green pharmacy." In addition, it is an easy, fun, and cheap hobby.

Aromatic herbs, in particular, are very good for a home garden since they are ideal for novice gardeners and they also reward you handsomely. Without investing much time or effort, they offer medicinal benefits and pleasant aroma, which you can use in multiple recipes or herbal remedies. They are versatile, ornamental, and fragrant. There are many possibilities from the wide range of varieties to choose from. Most go well in planters, but they will need more water and nutrients than if they are planted in soil. Rosemary, thyme, sage, oregano, marjoram, peppermint, basil, chives, or parsley are some herbs that you can plant at home.

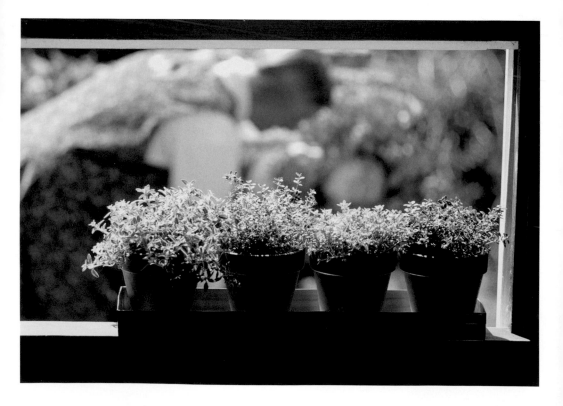

How to **select** the most suitable plant

To successfully grow plants, decide where you want to grow them, and select the most appropriate and healthy ones so you can plant them correctly. Get them at a good garden center or, better yet, in a specialized nursery, where you can get information and advice from knowledgeable staff. First, find strong plants, and avoid weak or decayed plants that have only a few stems and pale or discolored leaves. A healthy plant is one in which the leaves reach the base of the stem, it is compact, and it has a good shape. Make sure that they are not infested with insects. Check that its soil is dry, has not shrunk, nor separated from the sides of the pot. If you can see a clump of roots protruding from the base, it means that its roots are crowded, and it should have been changed into a much bigger pot long ago.

Transport

Once you have selected the right plant, be careful while taking it home, do not let it tip over and break. Do not leave it inside a hot and stuffy car for a long time, and water it well as soon as you get home. Plant it as soon as possible.

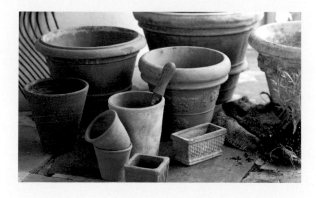

Annual plants are preferable

When choosing them, please note that annual plants are much easier to grow than biennial or perennial, since these last two have to be taken out of their pot and pruned to keep them in good condition. The most recommended in this regard would be basil, an annual plant that is easy to grow, much like thyme, rosemary, lavender, peppermint, or oregano.

It is still recommended that you switch aromatic plants into a larger pot every year or two. Multiply them by using their cuttings or seeds and let the new replace the old, and prune both roots and shoots.

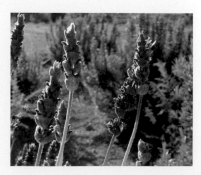

Where should you place them?

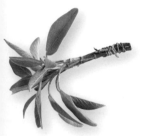

The dry and warm areas of the balcony, terrace, or garden are suitable for a wide variety of plants, because in general almost all of them do well in the sun. And as long as they get enough moisture in their roots, they should have no problem. This will work for thyme, lavender, angelica, celery, and caraway. Also, there are plants that prefer shade and whose appearance may worsen if they are exposed to direct sunlight throughout the day, for example, oregano, parsley, peppermint, sage, or lemon balm.

How much **water** do they need?

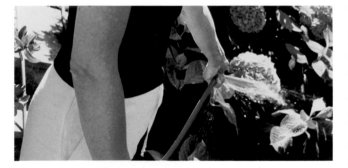

Many herbs are native to the Mediterranean climate (e.g., hyssop, lavender, lemon balm, oregano, sage, lavender cotton, thyme, rosemary), and as such they need little water to live. But there are some that need more moisture, such as peppermint and parsley, and you will have to water them frequently, even several times a day in summer if they get direct sunlight.

Keep in mind . . .

For optimum irrigation, it is important to note the following:

- It should be done using clean water, free of chemicals. Although each plant requires a certain periodicity, watering should be regular and even to avoid flooding, which can rot the roots and promote the spread of harmful fungi and bacteria.

- Drain it well by placing several pieces of pottery at the bottom of the planter.

- It is best to water the plant during the early hours of the morning or at dusk, rather than at the sunniest hours of the day.

- When they start to lose some freshness and vitality, water them well.

What should you **consider?**

Fertilizer

Herbs are fertilized very little so that they do not lose their flavor and aroma. They prefer soil with a normal amount of mineral nutrients.

Fertilize the soil once a year. Organic fertilizer (manure, compost, peat, etc.) is applied in winter, and in spring/fall if it contains minerals (or chemicals). You can use organic fertilizers such as guano, dry leaves, or compost. It is very important to use fertilizers from well-composted waste and to use only the recommended amount. Inadequately using fertilizers or using them in excessive amounts may leave residues on the ground that could be potentially hazardous to your health.

Pruning

Herbs like oregano, peppermint, lemon balm, lavender, or thyme have to be cut after they bloom to encourage healthy growth; otherwise, they will become woody. Come summer, cut plants such as peppermint to stimulate growth of new leaves. It is best to prune thyme a little and often throughout the spring and summer.

But even after you have pruned them every year, after a few years they will need to be uprooted and replaced with new ones as they often lose their original form.

Trim plants that have any overgrowth. Remove dead and dry parts of the plant, which eat up its nutrients and disfigure the plant.

Tarragon and peppermint spread rapidly by means of underground stems, which can invade surrounding plants, becoming "weeds." By planting them inside a buried planter, you will limit their lateral expansion. Another option is to cut them often so they do not become invasive.

Other care

Throughout the year, dig up the ground so as to break the surface, aerate the soil, squash it and pull out any weeds that may have grown around the plants. Till the very surface of the soil, without going in too deeply, as that could break roots. You should do this at least twice a year and up to five or six times.

Plants against pests

An infusion of basil, elderberry, or garlic with a teaspoon of mild detergent or soap will get rid of aphids. Some dried herbs, such as sage, can be sprinkled on plants to keep away slugs and snails.

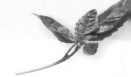

What if I need them for cooking?

Whenever you need a sprig of parsley or peppermint, cut off a stem using scissors, always above a bud, so that the plant can continue to grow.

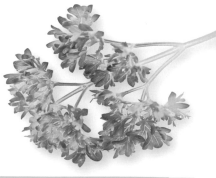

Some **plants** for your balcony

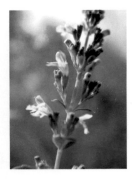

Summer savory
(Satureja hortensis)

This annual plant is currently widespread throughout the Mediterranean. It grows up to 10 inches (25 centimeters) and its leaves are soft, with a slightly rounded tip and covered with short hairs. The small flowers grow together in clusters.

It is an easy plant to grow in a very sunny place. It requires well-drained soil and little water, so you must water it only when the soil is very dry.

The flowering tops are harvested from late spring to early autumn. They are placed on paper and left to dry in a shady, well-ventilated place. Then they are stored in sealed containers. They can increase the production of gastric juice, which promotes digestion. They also have an antispasmodic effect, especially on the intestinal muscles, and work as an anti-diarrheic. Prepare an infusion by mixing a teaspoon of summer savory per cup of water to treat digestive disorders.

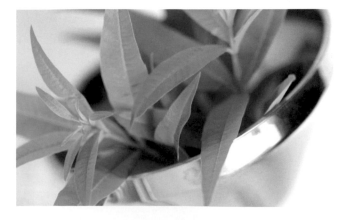

Lemon verbena
(Lippia citriodora)

Lemon verbena is a shrub that comes from South America and usually grows to 6.5 feet (2 meters) high, although in warm areas it can grow up to 13 feet (4 meters). Its elongated leaves are attached to the stem by a knot, grouped in three or four. Its pale purple or lilac flowers grow in clusters, and it blooms in summertime.

It can be grown in pots, but bear in mind that it prefers warm places and well-drained soil. It requires direct sun, and during the summer it needs frequent watering, practically every day. It does well when it gets fertilizer every two weeks. However, in winter it requires less irrigation but must be protected from frost. Remove any dried leaves and wilted flowers so that it can continue looking healthy.

Its leaves have a strong lemon scent that is used for culinary purposes. They are usually harvested during the summer, then dried and stored in tightly sealed containers. They also have medicinal value because they have digestive, antispasmodic, and sedative effects. For this reason, an infusion prepared by mixing a teaspoon of leaves per cup of water is very effective for calming the nerves, treating insomnia, and improving digestion.

Marjoram
(Origanum majorana)

This biennial or perennial plant is native to North Africa. It grows 2 feet (60 centimeters) high, and its oval leaves are of a color ranging from green to gray-green, depending on the abundance of hair. The delicate white, lilac, or purple flowers of this plant grow in thick clusters, making it a very decorative plant.

It can be easily grown in pots, but it does not do well in harsh winters. It needs direct sunlight and well-drained soil. Water it when its soil gets dry, early in the morning or at dusk. The flowering tops are harvested in summer then dried in a well-ventilated area (no more than 73°F [23°C]) and stored in tightly closed glass jars.

Marjoram has a strong and pleasant fragrance that is very appreciated in the kitchen. It also has medicinal uses to improve poor digestion due to its digestive and antispasmodic properties. It is also a good urinary antiseptic. It is most commonly used as a tea that is prepared by mixing one teaspoon of marjoram per cup of water. However, keep in mind that it is contraindicated during pregnancy and lactation, and for children under the age of twelve. Marjoram works as a fragrant insect repellent for your home.

Thyme
(Thymus vulgaris)

Thyme is a Mediterranean perennial plant that grows to 1.6 feet (50 centimeters) high. Its stem is stiff and woody with tiny leaves. The flowers, which range from white to purple, are rich in essential oil and give it its flavor and properties.

Its cultivation in pots is very easy because you only need to provide it a lot of sun. It grows well in all soil types, you do not need much water, and it even resists drought quite well. However, in summer you have to water it much more than the rest of the year. To drain it well, place shards of pottery in the bottom of the pot.

To use it fresh, cut tender stalks, separate the leaves, and finely chop it. To use it dry, cut its stems a few centimeters above the ground, just before the plant blooms. Once dry, the leaves are separated and stored in tightly closed containers.

Its culinary use is well known, but it also has medicinal properties. It alleviates some digestive disorders and has expectorant and antispasmodic effect, making it a useful remedy for colds, bronchitis, and dry cough. Make an infusion using a teaspoon of dried thyme, three times a day. Mix thyme with peppermint or rosemary, to make a poultice, and use it to relieve rheumatic pains. Use it in a decoction for its antiseptic effect to treat minor injuries. It can also be used as fragrance in your home. Place some of its twigs in indoor planters or add them to a potpourri, or you can even place them in cloth bags.

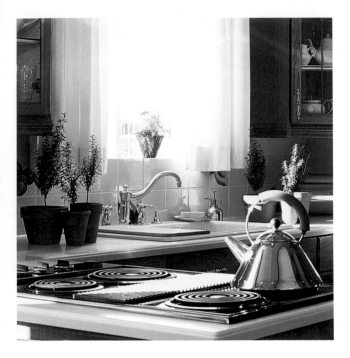

Their advantages

Aromatic plants cannot be regarded as nutritionally indispensable, since they generally only provide a small amount of fiber and minerals, but sparingly added to food, their aromatic and medicinal properties constitute the start of a good digestive process.

For starters, by enhancing the flavor of foods and making them more appetizing, they stimulate our appetite, prompting us to eat more, which is very important for those suffering from poor appetite. They increase digestive secretions (from saliva to intestinal juices) that are necessary for good digestion. And as if this were not enough, many of them, such as fennel, dill, and oregano, have a carminative effect, meaning that they help reduce or even prevent the production of annoying intestinal gas or flatulence.

Another virtue that they all share is that they are good substitutes for salt, which many times causes fluid retention, and that is especially not recommended for people with hypertension and many women. Herbs are also very good food preservatives, slowing or inhibiting the growth of microorganisms. This is attributed to the antiseptic, antimicrobial, and antifungal effect from their richness in essential oils. In short, besides being an undeniable part of international cuisine, herbs are not only palatable, but they are the perfect, healthy, and natural complement to any dish for a healthy diet.

From the earliest times, herbs have been known and used in magical and religious rituals, cosmetics, and perfumes. But they have always been giving culinary uses to try to vary and improve the monotonous flavor of everyday meals or even to disguise the bad taste of certain foods. Today, few dishes are made without one or more of these herbs as an ingredient. By themselves, they are not particularly good, but moderately and gracefully combined, they are able to make a bland or tasteless dish into something really appealing and tasteful, without masking its true flavor. And good nutrition begins with tasteful sensations.

How they are used in the kitchen

Herbs can be included in simple everyday dishes. All you need for a more varied and interesting menu is to add some twigs, sticks, or finely chopped fresh leaves, either from one single herb or by mixing multiple herbs.

Herbs are often shredded or crushed so that they can more easily release their aromatic substances. Although the amount to be added varies by taste, it is best to add them in small amounts until you are pleased with its taste. Do not use them in large amounts because instead of enhancing the basic taste of food, you risk dominating its flavor with the taste of herbs and ruining your meal.

Freshly cut herbs are highly recommended for their flavor, freshness, and especially for their health benefits; using them fresh is best, except for bay laurel, which is usually used dry. In general, use a tablespoon of chopped

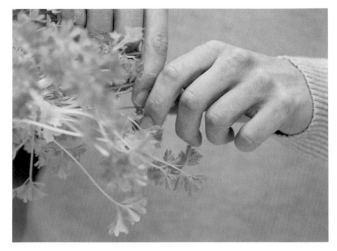

fresh herbs for four people. Dry herbs are more concentrated, so use a half or third of a spoonful to achieve the same effect. If they are fresh and you would rather remove them before serving, place them in a cloth bag. If they are twigs, tie them together with thread that you can pull out.

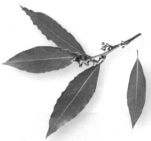

Aromatic blends

Many recipes typically include a bunch of different herbs as ingredients. Herbs for broths are wrapped in thin cloth to keep them gathered together, but herbs used in stews or casseroles are simply tied with a cord to release their aromas. Such herbal blends can be made with fresh and dried herbs. Different combinations and their use depends on individual taste, there are no rules, although there are certain traditional combinations that never fail. Some that give excellent results are as follows:

- Herbes de Provence: mix equal parts thyme, rosemary, basil, savory, and sometimes lavender. You can also add oregano, marjoram, and fennel to taste. Chop them fresh or dried.

- Fines herbes: it is a delicate blend of equal parts parsley, chervil, chives, and sometimes tarragon. These herbs are finely chopped, and they can also be used dry.

- Bouquet garni: there is no generic recipe for bouquet garni, but it commonly includes three sprigs of parsley, thyme, and a bay leaf. It works well if you wrap it around a celery stalk or the green part of a leek. Depending on the stew, you can also include basil, rosemary, savory, and tarragon.

Conservation

The flavor and aroma when herbs are fresh are incomparable, so if you have a sunny balcony, a terrace, or a garden patch, they are worth having. To use them regularly, you only need to cut off the leaves of the plant and make way for new growth. But if you do not have anywhere to grow them, get them fresh at the market where it is increasingly common to find them in sealed packages. Once you get them home, they can be kept in the refrigerator inside a sealed plastic bag or an

Some aromatic plants

● **Basil (*Ocimum basilicum*)**
Delicate and fragrant, the most common basil has light green leaves that are glossy and lance shaped. It is very easy to grow in pots or in the garden, which will allow you to use it fresh or dry. Its leaves and flowering tops have antispasmodic, digestive effect that can calm nervous disorders and migraines due to poor digestion. It also aids during menstruation and decreases menstrual cramps. Moreover, it is a tonic plant, which mitigates fatigue and nervous exhaustion. However, using its essential oil is not advisable since it may have a carcinogenic effect. Taken orally in high doses, it may have a narcotic effect. Applied externally in high doses, it can irritate the mucous membranes. Basil is particularly aromatic, with a fresh scent that resembles peppermint and pepper. Its

flavor is a combination of sweet and spicy, making it the ideal dressing for many dishes. It is used in salads and tomato sauces, and it is a basic ingredient for many pasta and vegetable dishes. To avoid losing its aroma, add when the food is done cooking.

● **Bay laurel (*Laurus nobilis*)**
Bay leaves come from a beautiful large tree. They are leathery and have an intense flavor and a pungent odor, which becomes more intense when it is dried. In herbal medicine its essential oil is for external use only; its rubefacient effect works as an anti-inflammatory and anti-rheumatic. It significantly relieves rheumatic and muscular pains. Adding its dried leaves to food stimulates appetite, digestive secretions, and intestinal functioning, which facilitate digestion. It is

indispensable in Mediterranean cuisine as a key condiment in vegetable stews, seafood broths, marinades, and brines. Its essential oil is very powerful so it should be used sparingly, and its leaves should never be crushed; simply take one or two and add them to the stew. Once you have cooked the dish, remove the leaves, because they retain their harsh texture and bitter aftertaste. Use them sparingly, otherwise they can be toxic. During pregnancy and lactation do not exceed the normal amounts for cooking.

● **Oregano (*Origanum vulgare*)**
Oregano is a perennial plant measuring about three palms in height. Its flowers bloom between July and September. And since there is nothing better than fresh oregano, try to always have some in the gar-

airtight container for six to seven days. Dry them or freeze them so you will have them available throughout the winter months.

Freezing

To freeze your herbs, make bouquets with one or more herbs, tie them, and spread them out on a tray. Once frozen, save them in a container to keep them from breaking. You may also want to chop them before preserving them. This way you have specific amounts set aside in packets, or place them in an ice cube tray where you will then make ice cubes. Once the ice cubes are ready, place them in another container for storage. Frozen herbs should be stored no longer than six months. Frozen herbs also retain their essential oils and color better than dry herbs.

Drying

To dry your herbs, tie them in bundles, wrap them in paper, and hang them upside down for ten to fifteen days in a dry, dark, and well-ventilated place. Once dried, chop them up on a large and clean piece of paper, remove the stems, and store them in clean and dry glass jars with lids. Keep the jars away from light and moisture.

den or in a pot. It can grow leaves and flowers for five or six years, then it is better to uproot it and replace it with a new one. It can be cut with scissors or close to the ground with flowers and all, because it will sprout again without any problem. Its leaves have a warm, slightly spicy, and very aromatic flavor. But they also have expectorant, cough suppressant, and slightly sedative effects. An infusion of oregano relieves coughing and insomnia. It also has antispasmodic and carminative properties, so when used as a condiment, it is a good remedy for nervous indigestion.

It is a fundamental plant in Italian and Greek cuisine, it is used to flavor meat, vegetables, and legumes, as well as develop digestive aromatic wines. It is also used in soups and to marinate meat for sausages.

Try sautéing some vegetables with a little extra virgin olive oil, garlic, and oregano to give them a surprising amount of flavor. And it also goes great with tomato sauce.

Although dry oregano is not comparable to fresh oregano, it retains its potency for a year.

● Parsley **(Petroselinum crispum)**
All parts of the parsley have the same fresh aroma, but undoubtedly the stems have greater intensity. Its leaves are set apart and have a strong green color, and they are most commonly used, whole or finely chopped. It is the most popular of all herbs used to decorate and flavor foods, but it is also rich in antioxidants, works like a diuretic, makes you hungry, stimulates menstruation, and it is invigorating. Both its infusion and fresh juice are good for edema or fluid retention, as well as during convalescence. Chew it after eating garlic, to prevent bad breath. Fresh and crushed leaves can be applied in poultices for wounds to heal more quickly and easily and to relieve pain from insect bites. It is always better fresh, so try growing it in your garden or in a pot. If these options are not available to you, buy it at the market. Its mild flavor and its ability to enhance the aroma of other herbs make it an indispensable element in classic blends. Given that its flavor is much more intense when raw than when it is fried or baked, add it after your food is done cooking. Finely chopped parsley on top of a dish is often used as an attractive green garnish.

To benefit from all its virtues, use parsley frequently and abundantly. It is a highly recommended herb for all, except during pregnancy and for those suffering from kidney stones, due to their abundance of oxalic acid.

IN THE BATHROOM

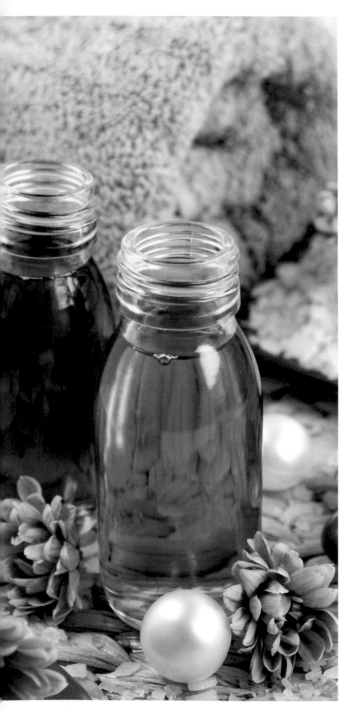

In addition to their medicinal effect, plants are great sources of health and beauty. Since ancient times they have been used to enhance female beauty or to prepare relaxing baths. In ancient Egypt, for example, perfumed baths were used for centuries with natural ingredients like myrrh, saffron, and cinnamon. In Greece, meanwhile, it was customary to entertain guests with a bath of lilies, roses, and almonds. And later, the Romans created public baths (hot springs) where it was common to use susinun, an ointment prepared with aromatic reeds, honey, cinnamon, saffron, and myrrh.

A good bath consists of natural products without chemical compounds, that is, the removal of excessive fat, which contributes to dry skin. Ideally, rather than using a gel or lotion with natural ingredients, add medicinal plants to bath water by pouring infusions or essential oils (aromatherapy). Herbs can nourish the skin, protect it against infection, and encourage its regeneration. In addition, they offer many benefits of aromatherapy because as we bathe in essences, their aromas travel up the nose, into the lungs, the circulatory system, and brain. Aromatherapy is a warm and pleasant technique to treat emotional problems, but it is better that you consult a therapist because there can be different reactions to the same scent.

Add an **herbal infusion** to water

Some medicinal plants are particularly beneficial as infusions added to bath water. Water will take on the herb's properties.

Poppy *(Papaver rhoeas)*
For its relaxing and soothing properties, it is ideal for preparing baths to alleviate circulatory problems.

Dandelion
(Taraxacum officinale)
The fresh plant is very rich in vitamin A and is ideal for its cleansing properties.

Golden everlasting
(Helichrysum bracteatum)
Considered a very valuable plant for skin care, it can be used to prepare nourishing and healing baths.

Linden flower *(Tilia cordata)*
Linden flower contains mucilage and essential oil, which are very good for improving and hydrating skin.

Also in the shower

To benefit from essential oils, you do not have to prepare a bath. If you do not have a bathtub or you are short in time, you can have aromatherapy in the shower. Although the results are not as effective, they always help, especially as toning and stimulating treatments.

Add essential oils to a wet washcloth or a sponge, run it through hot water and scrub your body vigorously, avoiding more sensitive areas. Two or three drops should be enough. You can also add eight drops of essential oil to your washcloth and place it on the showerhead, and when you open the tap, deeply inhale the vapors released by the hot water.

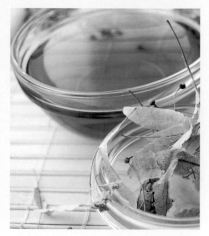

Keep in mind . . .

You can also prepare infusions with different plants and create baths for different purposes:

- Relaxing bath:
  Prepare an infusion by mixing 3 tablespoons of sage with 3 tablespoons of lavender, and then strain it in hot bath water. Soaking in this bath for 15 or 20 minutes, relaxes and helps calm tensions.

- Stimulating bath:
  Place 3 tablespoons (50 grams) of rosemary and 3 tablespoons (50 grams) of rose petals in 4 cups (1 liter) of boiling water. Cover it and let simmer for 10 minutes. Strain the infusion and pour it into your bath water. Lastly, add a few drops of lemon essential oil and proceed to enjoy an energizing bath.

Add a little **pouch** with plants to your bath water

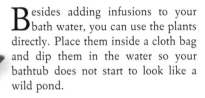

Besides adding infusions to your bath water, you can use the plants directly. Place them inside a cloth bag and dip them in the water so your bathtub does not start to look like a wild pond.

Soaps with plants

These are essential and can be easily made at home with products you find at the grocery store. They give amazing results that are far better than commercial products you find in the health and beauty aisles of any store. Normally, soap is manufactured by mixing caustic soda and fat because their mixture causes "saponification." However, you can also make soaps without caustic soda by using a glycerin soap base, which is great for skin care. Shredded, grated soap can also be used as a base. Add leaves, flowers, petals, or the roots of medicinal plants such as chamomile or rosemary, as well as essential oils such as rose. Here's an example:

Herbal soap

Prepare an infusion by mixing rosemary, peppermint, and chamomile, and set aside half a glass. Place it in a double boiler, then grate and add a bar of pure conventional soap, which will start to melt while you stir the mixture. When it has a creamy, thick consistency, remove it from heat and pour it into a plastic container. Take it out of the mold after a couple of days, and wrap the soap in paper to protect it.

Flower bath

- 1 cup (100 grams) lavender
- ½ cup (50 grams) bitter orange peel
- 1 tablespoon of each: thyme, wild rose leaves, willow, borage, peppermint, marjoram, rosemary
- 2 cloves, chopped
- A few drops of lemon
- 5 drops of rose essential oil

Mix the lavender and orange peel with the other plants, then add the two cloves, lemon drops, and rose oil. Place everything in a cloth bag, tie it shut, and place it in the bathtub under warm running water. This bath will soften sensitive skin that tends to chafe.

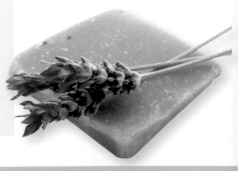

Mix a few drops of **essential oil** in water

In hot or cold bath water, essential oils penetrate through pores of the skin. Furthermore, water vapor releases active ingredients in essential oils, and you inhale them into your respiratory tract and brain through the nose. Science has now shown and reaffirmed what Hippocrates already knew in the 4th century BC: taking a daily aromatic bath is good for the body and soul. These essential oils that are rich in active ingredients and fragrances are the basis for aromatherapy.

About six drops are enough for a scented bath, but you may use more for a healing effect on the body or emotions. In this case, you should seek advice from an aroma therapist, and you should not exceed the recommended amount. Avoid getting it in your eyes, because they might get a little irritated. Once you have chosen an essential oil, add it to the water and mix it, then get in the water right away to make the most of its active ingredients; it evaporates quickly due to the high temperature of the water.

As essential oils dissolve only in fat, it is normal to see small droplets distributed throughout the water. Try mixing essential oils in a cup of milk where they will dissolve well, then add the milk to the bath water. This aromatherapy technique was used by Cleopatra, who was famous for taking baths in donkey's milk.

Tips for preparing a bath

- Create a warm and welcoming atmosphere in the bathroom with soothing music, soft lighting, candles. . . .
- Do not take longer than twenty minutes; staying longer can affect your heart and circulatory system. Your skin will swell and lose its protective acid coating.
- The water temperature should not exceed 96.8°F (36°C), because if it is too hot, the bath loses its calming effect.
- Two or three baths a week are sufficient to achieve the desired effect, anything else is just excessive.
- After a relaxing bath, wait a while before engaging in any activity that requires alertness such as driving. Ideally, take the bath right before bedtime at the end of a long day.
- Besides essential oils or herbal infusions, you can add Dead Sea salt, which has many properties, to prepare a calming bath.
- If you want to soothe muscular pain, treat depression, etc., take a good shower first and then soak in the tub with hot water and essential oils only. Soap, vegetable oil, or bath salts do not let the pores absorb these active ingredients adequately.

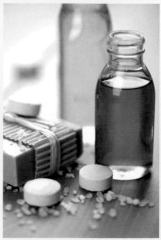

The best **oils** for the bath

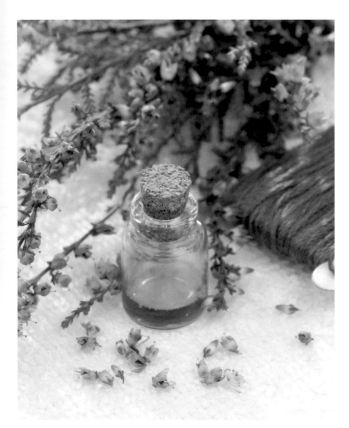

or simply inhale the aroma when you need to feel lively or if you are suffering from insomnia.

An evening bath with ylang-ylang oil helps eliminate daily tensions and restore calm and balance. In aromatherapy, ylang-ylang is one of the most relaxing fragrances for the mind and the body. It also lowers blood pressure slightly and acts as a natural antidepressant. However, studies show that the scent is both stimulating and relaxing to brain waves; much like other natural remedies, it seems to energize or calm, depending on the individual's needs. It is also very effective when mixed with sweet almond oil and applied before shampooing to treat split ends and dandruff.

Dog-rose
(*Rosa canina*)

Dog-rose is well known for its aroma, and its essence is very beneficial when used for massage, bath, or inhalation. Thirty roses are used for making a single drop of essence.

Its therapeutic action is very broad. Externally, it can be used as an ophthalmic and to treat skin problems. The pharmaceutical industry uses more red rose petals than white rose petals, due to their higher tannin content that has a slightly astringent action; for this reason they are preferred for eye drops and chronic eye diseases.

Ylang-ylang
(*Cananga odorata*)

The essence of ylang-ylang is used in skin treatments to hydrate and reduce excess sebum. Add it to your bath, mix it with sweet almond oil for massage,

It is also one of the most antiseptic essences. Its slightly tonic and soothing qualities, and its effect on the capillaries, make it suitable for almost all skin types, especially for mature, dry, or sensitive skin, and for redness or swelling. It also acts on the nervous system externally or by inhalation, relaxing and promoting sleep. Internally, it is beneficial for the female genital area, and it has circulatory and digestive properties (nausea and vomiting).

Winter jasmine
(Jasminum nudiflorum)

The essence of jasmine acts as anti-inflammatory, antiseptic, muscle relaxant, analgesic, and expectorant. On an emotional level, it is considered a powerful natural antidepressant and can produce feelings such as optimism and euphoria. Simply detecting its scent awakens an emotional state of greater confidence and serenity. Given that many sexual problems are caused by stress, anxiety, or fear, the scent of jasmine is ideal for relieving them. Create a pleasant and special atmosphere by placing it on the stove, and use it for an aromatic bath. For massage, mix seven drops of jasmine oil and half a cup of almond oil, which provides a nice warm and relaxing effect.

Bergamot
(Citrus bergamia)

Bergamot is a citrus fruit from southern Italy. You could say it is a small orange that has a fresh scent like most citrus. Its peel is used to extract greenish yellow essential oil that has a sweet and sour flavor with interesting properties, most notably its antidepressant effect. Bergamot essence creates a very pleasant atmosphere that can help reduce anxiety and depression, which can be attributed to its stimulating effect. Externally, it also heals and works like an antiseptic. It is widely used in fragrances, especially in men's colognes. Infusions are also prepared and added to edible products. At home it can be used in oil burners or soaps. Mix a few drops of essential oil, water, and alcohol and spray your pillow or keep a handkerchief sprayed with bergamot in your purse to sniff whenever you need it. It is a very special gift for anyone who may be going through a difficult situation.

Geranium
(Pelargonium graveolens)

Geranium is a known insect repellent, and it is used in the cosmetics industry. Its essential oil is very useful for skin care due to its ability to balance sebum production. It also has an antiseptic and antibacterial effect, so gargling with two or three drops in a glass of water will relieve sore throats and help heal mouth sores. Because of its diuretic and stimulating effect on the lymphatic system, geranium also helps the body eliminate fluids. On an emotional aspect, it promotes harmony and emotional balance by dispelling negative thoughts and feelings of unease and anxiety.

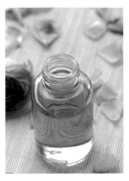

IN THE BOUDOIR

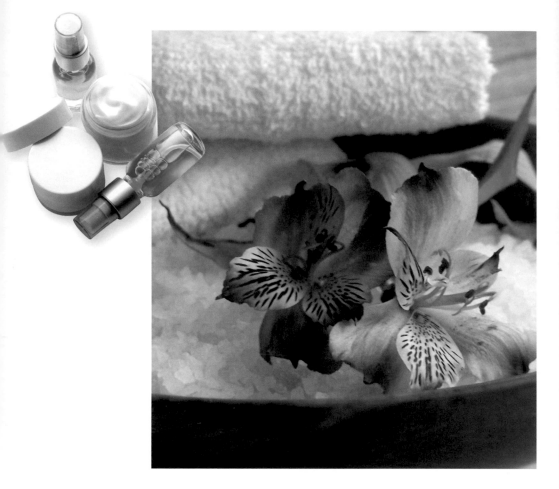

To feel beautiful, you do not need to spend a lot of time or spend a lot of money on cosmetics. By daily using certain ingredients that nature offers us, you can enhance your own beauty. Of course, every body part has its own needs and requires specific care. Here you will find the best natural treatments to pamper your skin, hair, hands, and your entire body and learn how to make your own beauty products at home. You will see that making your own personal care products brings a unique element of pleasure. But do not forget that to feel beautiful on the outside you must also take care of yourself from within.

Soothing tonic

- 1 tablespoon of chamomile
- 1 ¼ cups (250 milliliters) of water

Make a chamomile infusion and let it steep for 5 minutes. Strain it and let it come to room temperature. For a calming and decongestant effect on the skin, soak a cotton ball in this infusion and dab it lightly on the skin.

Show off your skin

Cleanliness is the first step in maintaining a healthy, luminous complexion. Cleansing your skin correctly every day will remove dust, make-up, and dirt, and it will unclog your sebaceous glands, preventing the appearance of pimples and blackheads. Lather your face using a shaving brush, rinse with warm water, pat it dry with a towel, then apply a tonic lotion. The cleanser you use will vary depending on your skin type: use a cream if you have dry skin, for example one made with avocado; for oily skin, use a gel, for example one made with cucumber. Then comes hydration, whose main mission is to restore the moisture your skin loses, by using vitamins, minerals, and trace elements. And do not forget using night or regenerative nourishing creams. Besides this daily care, you can improve your complexion by doing the following on a weekly basis: exfoliating and

applying face masks. Exfoliating once a week can renew the epidermis, cleanse, and gently remove dead cells and impurities. After exfoliating, your face is ready for a mask that must meet three requirements: be unctuous, be sticky enough, and can be easily removed. Banana, avocado, honey, eggs, yogurt, wheat germ, even lettuce, are some of the ingredients in your pantry that you can use to make simple and effective cosmetics.

Lotion to diminish oiliness

- 3 teaspoons chopped peppermint
- 2 teaspoons cider vinegar
- 4 cups (1 liter) distilled water

Place peppermint and cider vinegar in a jar, close it well, and let it marinate for at least one week, then filter it and add distilled water.

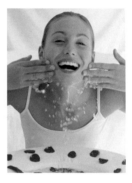

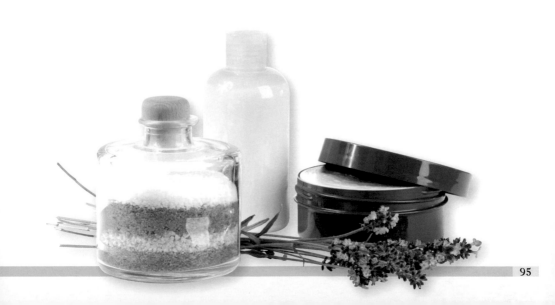

Caring for **eyes and lips**

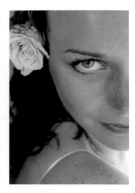

When cleaning your face, be careful with the contour of your eyes because its surrounding skin is very thin and delicate. Use a specific makeup-removing product to prevent an allergic reaction. To apply, use a cotton ball and move it gently down the upper eyelids and eyelashes, toward the inner corner of the eye. Then use a cream or gel for bags under your eyes, dark circles, or crow's feet; apply it by gently tapping with your fingertips, both morning and evening. A very simple trick to get rid of puffy eyes is to boil some water with coarse salt, soak a cotton ball in it, and keep it on the eye area for ten minutes. Calming herbal products such as marigold, mallow, or

Marigold lip cream

To soften and moisturize your lips, make an infusion of marigold, strain it, and let it cool off, then melt a tablespoon of shea butter in a small container using a double boiler, add a tablespoon of apricot oil, then add the infusion. Place it inside a jar, close it, and shake well to emulsify the mixture. Let the cream cool before using.

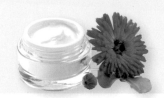

chamomile are effective at reducing tightness caused by fatigue.

Just as with the eyes, lips need special care. Lacking oil glands, lips tend to dry out and crack, especially with the cold and wind, so they require extra protection. Try using a moisturizing lip balm throughout the day. A good natural remedy is to coat them with honey and then rub them gently with a slice of avocado, or massage them with a few drops of olive oil before bedtime.

Apply tea

One way to relax your eyes and prevent swelling is to make tea and store the drained bags in the refrigerator. Then place them on your eyelids and leave them on for a few minutes while you relax.

Soothe your eyes with chamomile

To relieve tired eyes, brew some tea using fennel, parsley, and chamomile (the latter is regarded as one of the best medicinal plants to soothe, relax, and reduce swelling in the eyes). When the infusion is warm, apply it on your eyes as a compress.

Best shampoos for the **hair**

The hair requires as much attention as the skin, but we often neglect it and limit ourselves to washing it with any shampoo, whether or not it is suitable for our hair type. Just as with the face, it is important for you to know whether your hair is oily, dry, or normal, because its care will vary accordingly. As a general recommendation, wash it with warm water, not too hot, and apply shampoo by massaging in a circular motion. Do not worry about the amount of foam it generates, as some of the purest and best shampoos do not foam at all. If they are made with yogurt, egg yolk, rosemary, and sage, even better. Applying cider vinegar before rinsing it off will leave your hair glossy. Apply a conditioner once a week for dry hair, every fifteen days for normal hair, and no more than once a month for oily hair. Finally, try not to use your hair drier every day, but rather let it air dry whenever possible. Trim the ends of your hair at least once every two months, and use brushes and combs with natural bristles to prevent damage. Replace chemical hair dyes with natural ones, such as henna, which contains no ammonia and other harsh substances.

Rosemary shampoo for oily hair

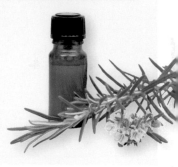

- 1 tablespoon neutral shampoo
- 1 egg yolk
- 3 drops of rosemary essential oil

Mix the ingredients well and beat them until forming a creamy paste. Shampoo your hair as you would normally. Do not save any remaining shampoo since it does not keep well.

Sage shampoo with proteins

- ⅜ cup (30 grams) sage
- 4 cups (1 liter) of water
- 1 cup neutral shampoo
- 2 eggs

Make an infusion of sage and strain it. Then heat it up and add dissolved soap in it, as you stir. Once cool, add the eggs and mix. Bottle it and let it steep for a whole day. Shake before using.

Softer **body**

Basil body oil

- 2 handfuls of basil flowers
- 4 cups (1 liter) of almond oil

Marinate the basil flowers in the oil for a month, and be sure that they are completely covered and do not protrude. Then filter the oil and remove the flowers to prevent them from rotting. This oil will retain the fragrance of fresh basil for many months.

Medicinal plants also provide skin care for the whole body. They pleasantly hydrate, soften, and nourish when used as creams, lotions, body oils, or added to bath water (discussed elsewhere in this chapter).

Rose body milk

- 8 cups (2 liters) of rosewater
- 1 ¼ cups (250 milliliters) infusion of rosemary
- 2 tablespoons of benzoin tincture
- ½ teaspoon of rose essential oil

Mix rose water with rosemary infusion, stirring constantly, and add benzoin. Finally, add the essential oil as a fragrance.

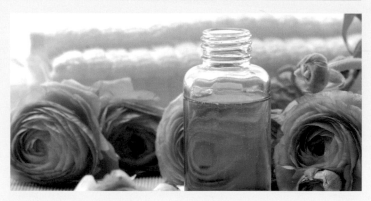

No trace of cellulite

The area comprising legs, abdomen, and buttocks is most prone to cellulite. This is due to the accumulation of fat, toxins, and water. Fat cells are enlarged and deformed until they become visible on the upper layers of the skin: unsightly skin that looks like an orange peel. This condition, as many others, must be fought on several fronts: diet, exercise, medicinal plants, and, of course, baths, creams, poultices, and masks are to be consistently applied externally on the affected areas. The most effective natural formulas are those that contain caffeine, ivy extract, ginkgo biloba extract, various algae, birch leaves, or horse chestnut, to name a few. It is also recommended to massage with aromatic oils such as lemon, juniper, orange, and cypress that have proven anti-cellulite properties.

Hands and feet like new

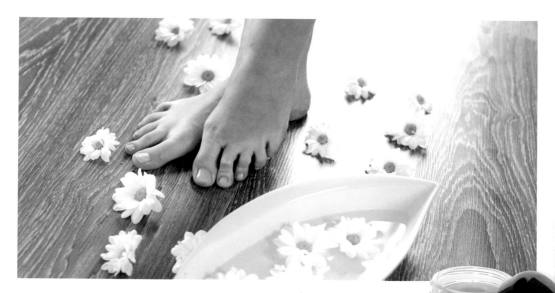

Hands are exposed to all weather conditions, water, soaps, and detergents, so it is no wonder that they show more signs of aging and neglect than other parts of the body that remain mostly protected. It is important to wash your hands with gentle soaps, made with natural ingredients such as coconut or almonds. Soaps with a high alkaline content tend to deteriorate the skin's natural pH, which is slightly acid, and cause dryness, roughness, and redness. So it is important to hydrate daily using a natural cream with cocoa butter or almond oil. Apply it at night with a gentle massage and wear cotton gloves overnight, then you will see the result in the morning. Cut and file your nails regularly, and do not bite them. Clean them, strengthen them, and rub them with lemon peel to bring out or restore their natural color. Winter is the time when hands suffer the most, and summer is a delicate time for feet, due to excessive sweating, tiredness, and heaviness, and, since you are not wearing socks, stockings, or boots, you will want them looking great in sandals. The most important thing is good hygiene: wash your feet daily, especially between the toes, and make sure you towel off any moisture that could cause fungus. Remember to gently scrub your feet to soften them and remove dead skin. Finally, hydrate and massage your feet with shea butter or avocado oil to keep them healthy and beautiful.

Some interesting **plants** for your boudoir

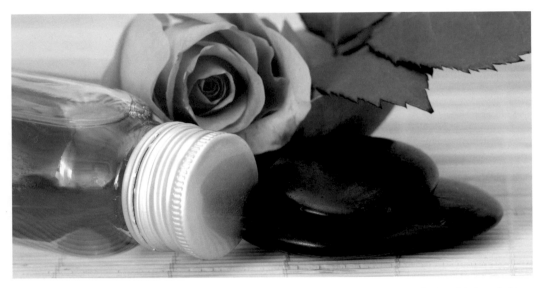

Avocado
(Persea americana)

Native to Mexico and Guatemala, avocado had been grown well before the arrival of the Spaniards. This delicacy nourishes and beautifies your skin and hair, whether you apply it directly or use its oil. To extract its oil, avocados are left to ripen until they look rotten, then they are boiled in water, and the excess oil is collected with a spoon then filtered to remove any impurities. Its oil is applied by rubbing it on the skin or scalp. Used externally, it stimulates the formation of collagen, which makes it a good balm for the skin, ideal for treating eczema or cracked and irritated skin. For youthful, supple, and wrinkle-free skin, apply an avocado face mask half an hour before bedtime. You can also use its oil. These same remedies can be used to treat pimples and blemishes and to prevent stretch marks during pregnancy. Avocado's softening and moisturizing properties make it a common ingredient in many creams for skin and hair care.

Sweet briar
(Rosa rubiginosa)

Its oil has a beautiful color ranging from yellowish orange to reddish, with a pleasant, mild aroma of the seeds from which it is obtained.

It is worth noting its content of natural tretinoin that has regenerative effect for the skin, as well as its unique richness in polyunsaturated essential fatty acids for its use in cosmetics. Its regenerating action works effectively against stretch marks and heals dehydrated and dry skin of all types. For example, pregnant women can use it to gently massage their breasts and abdomen during the last trimester of pregnancy to prevent stretch marks. After using it, their skin will be smoother, it will feel fresh, and it will have a new visible sheen. It also helps reduce the appearance of wrinkles, lines, burns, and scars and gives good results as treatment for psoriasis.

Marshmallow
(Althaea officinalis)
The most interesting part of the marshmallow is its root, which is rich in mucilage, although its leaves and flowers are also used. When used internally, marshmallow calms coughing, works as a laxative, and has a slight hypoglycemic effect (lowers glucose levels). Due to its ability to retain water in its mucilage, its use is very beneficial for treating dry skin, which needs more water to improve its texture, consistency, brightness, and vitality. It also has an anti-inflammatory and calming effect, so it is used for boils and eczema, as well as to relieve insect bites. Crush some leaves and use its juice to make compresses that you apply on the affected area.

Sesame oil
(Sesamum indicum)
This oil is extracted from cold-pressed sesame seeds. Buy it unrefined so you can fully benefit from all its acti-

ve ingredients. It revitalizes the skin against sagging. It is also very useful as a hair mask for excessive dryness or scabs on the scalp. In recent years, it is being studied for its effectiveness as a sunscreen to protect from UVB rays. In summertime, it also helps you get a natural tan and keeps your skin moisturized.

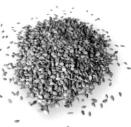

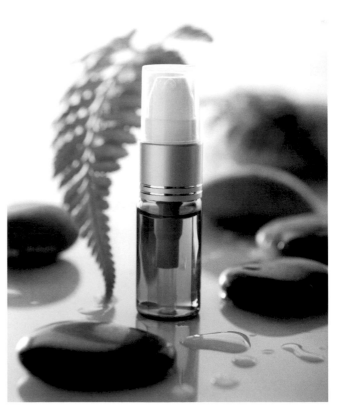

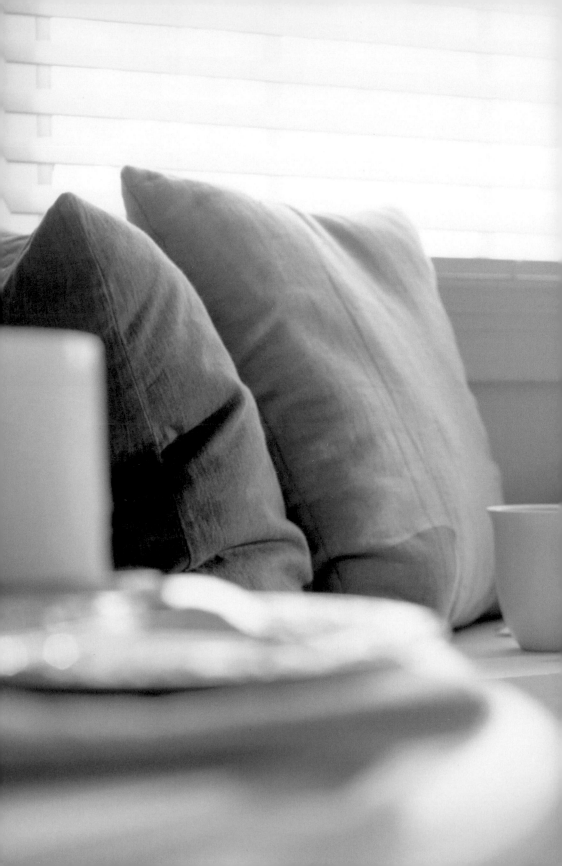

For your health

The many effects

Relaxing

At some point in our lives, we all experience nervousness, irritability, stress—even depression or anxiety. Fortunately, nature has given us some medicinal plants with sedative effect that are perfect for relaxing and restoring balance.

Revitalizing

Against tiredness and fatigue, common to modern life, there are herbs that have a tonic effect on our central nervous system or give us support in especially difficult times.

Anti-inflammatory (anti-rheumatic)

There is growing interest in using medicinal plants to treat various inflammatory reactions, in particular rheumatism, because they offer several advantages over common anti-inflammatory medications, including a lower incidence of negative side effects. Medicinal plants are particularly beneficial for older adults.

Respiratory

Ranging from the common cold to bronchitis, respiratory diseases are among the most common illnesses for people of all ages. To treat them, you can use medicinal plants with pectoral activity, whose effect is usually longer lasting and their side effects are fewer compared to some drugs.

Digestive

Digestive disorders can easily happen through changing mealtimes, unbalanced diet, stress—and they cause bloating, indigestion, flatulence, or constipation. To treat them, there is a wide range of medicinal plants that stimulate appetite, have a carminative effect (facilitate the expulsion of gas), and stimulate gastric secretions.

Circulatory

Nature provides us with a number of medicinal plants that tone and strengthen veins and arteries, improving blood circulation. For this reason, they can be used for treating such common disorders as varicose veins and hemorrhoids, among other circulatory problems that often affect us.

Liver

In addition to following a healthy diet that includes avoiding excesses, toxic substances, and alcohol abuse, using medicinal plants to stimulate liver functions significantly helps improve digestion, which is often affected when the liver is not functioning as it should.

Kidneys

Urinary tract infection, fluid retention, and kidney stones are some kidney disorders that can be treated effectively by using medicinal plants that have diuretic and purifying action. Drinking plenty of water between meals is also good for your health.

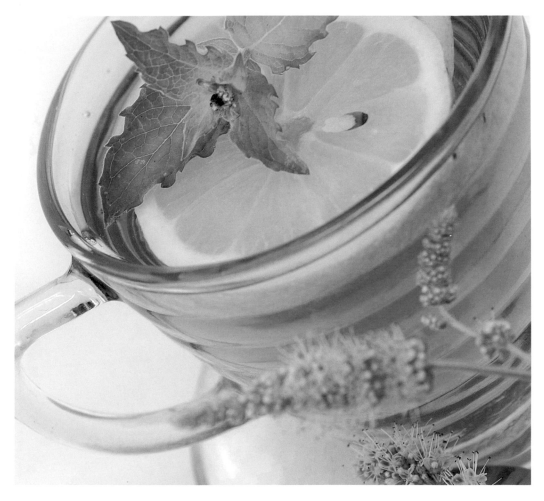

For the skin

Using plants to maintain or beautify the skin is a very old tradition. Their moisturizing, emollient, and healing properties are really effective to cure and care without any harshness.

Immunostimulators

Medicinal plants can be used to prevent the onset of winter infections, help during convalescence, or to keep children and older adults healthier by stimulating the immune system, which is responsible for the body's defenses against infections and other diseases. They are the most natural way to prevent the flu, colds, and other typical illnesses.

For the eyes and mouth

For common problems, such as a toothache or conjunctivitis, nature puts at our disposal a series of medicinal plants. On the following pages, you will find the three most commonly used and safe medicinal plants to treat such problems.

Golden poppy

(Eschscholzia californica)

Facilitates natural, restful sleep

Also known as cup of gold, it is native to California, where it was traditionally used by Native Americans as an analgesic and its sedative applications became popular among the rural population in California. It was brought to Europe in the 19th century as an ornamental plant.

When should you use it?

California poppy has a notable sedative, hypnotic effect and induces sleep, decreases the time it takes to fall asleep, has a calming effect when taken before bedtime, and improves quality of sleep. It is a good remedy for initial insomnia, but it is not as effective for staying asleep throughout the night. It is not addictive nor does it leave you feeling drowsy in the morning.

It is also a good anxiolytic for emotional stress and anxiety, and it eases nervousness and irritation both in adults and children. This plant also has some antidepressant effect and, thanks to its antispasmodic properties, it is recommended for muscle cramps that can wake you up at night. Finally, its sedative effect relieves itchy hives.

Presentation

It is most commonly found as capsules filled with the micronized powder from the plant's dried flower tops. The recommended dosage for an adult is one to two capsules (depending on the manufacturer) three times a day. The capsules can be taken with a glass of water and the last dose is best taken half an hour before bedtime.

Remedies

BY ITSELF

The easiest and safest way to take it is in capsules, but its infusion is also effective for relieving gastrointestinal spasms associated with stressful situations.

COMBINED

Infusion for sleeping: mix equal parts California poppy, passion flower, and lemon balm. Boil a spoonful of this mixture in a cup of water and let it sit. Drink it hot, before bedtime.

Infusion for itching: place a teaspoon of California poppy and a teaspoon of peppermint in a cup, add boiling water and let it steep for ten minutes. Apply it to the skin using a cotton ball once the infusion is lukewarm.

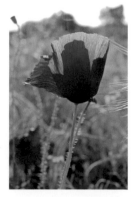

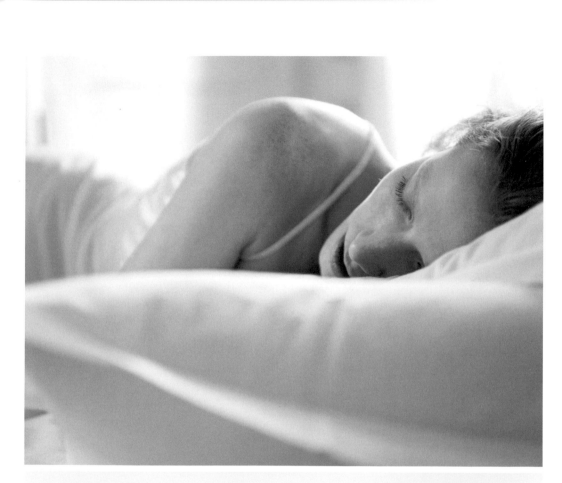

Precautions
Do not use during pregnancy and lactation, or for glaucoma, as it may increase intraocular pressure. Use it with caution if you are driving because it can cause drowsiness. It should not be administered along with other sedatives, as it could enhance relaxation.

Description
It is a perennial and annual herbaceous plant. Its leaves grow out of its stems, and its large cup-like flowers close at night and when it is not sunny. Its color ranges from yellow to red, depending on the variety.

Cultivation
It is native to the dry and sandy soil of California, but it has managed to adapt to European soil where it is grown for both ornamental and medicinal purposes.

Harvesting
The usable part of the plant grows above ground, and it is collected when it is in bloom.

Composition
The California poppy has alkaloids, flavonoids, cyanogenic glycosides, and carotenes.

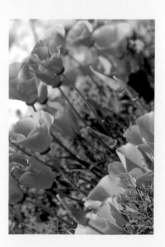

Hawthorn

(Crataegus monogyna)

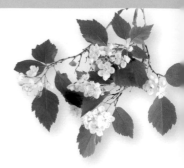

Tones the heart and calms the nerves

In ancient Greece, it was believed that hawthorn had an invigorating effect for goats, hence its scientific name, *Crataegus*, i.e., "strong goats." But the ancient Greeks also considered hawthorn a symbol of protection and purity, so it was placed in the marriage bed and in cribs to expel evil spirits.

When should you use it?

It has been called "valerian of the heart" because of its anxiolytic effect (eliminates anxiety), antispasmodic effect, and its strong cardiotonic action by which it is able to regulate heart rate and reduce arrhythmias. This makes it one of the most effective remedies for anxiety, nervousness, and stress, tightness in the chest, difficulty breathing, rapid heartbeat, or palpitations. It is especially suitable to treat insomnia. This plant works like a diuretic, and it is useful for regulating blood pressure.

Presentation

You can buy the dried and chopped plant by weight or in teabags, in capsules, and liquid extract (drops). It is also often found in combination with other sedative plants such as valerian and linden flower to treat stress, anxiety, and other nervous disorders. These combinations are sold in teabags and tablets. It is very important that whenever you buy any of these products, you read the instructions carefully so you take the proper dose.

Remedies

BY ITSELF

Infusion to reduce anxiety: place a teaspoon of crushed dried and ground hawthorn (troches) in a cup and add boiling water. Let it steep for ten minutes and strain it. Sweeten it with sugar or honey and drink up to three cups a day.

COMBINED

Infusion for sleeping: mix equal parts hawthorn, orange blossom, passionflower, and linden. Place a teaspoon of this mixture in a cup of boiling water. After ten minutes, strain it and drink it warm half an hour before bedtime. If you take three cups throughout the day, it can also work against anxiety.

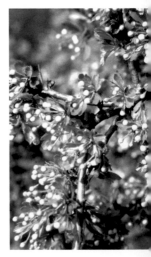

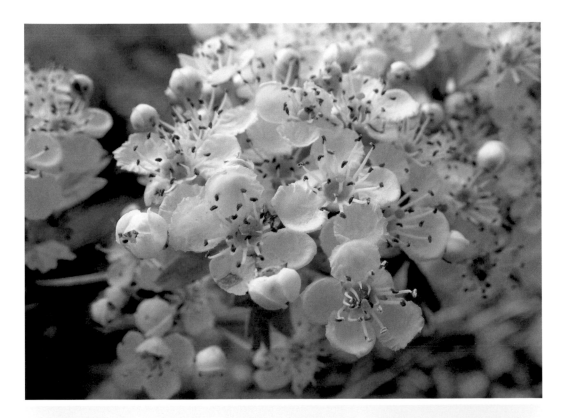

Precautions
It should not be administered to children under the age of twelve or women who are pregnant or breastfeeding. Only use it with medical supervision if you suffer from hypertension or coronary disease, and if you are taking other medications (especially digitalis).

Description
It is a thorny shrub that grows to 6 to 12 feet (2 to 4 meters) high. Its leaves are deciduous with a bright beam. Its white flowers are small and fragrant. Its berries (fruit) are red and edible.

Cultivation
It is common in European forests, but it is also found throughout America. It grows wild in streams and hillsides, embankments, and edges of farmland.

Harvesting
Its leaves, flowers, and fruits are used. Its leaves and flowers are harvested between May and July, and its fruit from September to October. It should be dried quickly in the shade and then stored in an airtight container in a cool, dark place.

Composition
Its chemical composition includes flavonoids, tannins, triterpenes, steroids, amines, and essential oil.

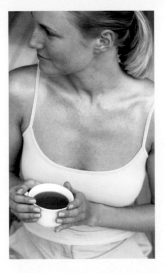

Lavender

(Lavandula angustifolia)

Its unmistakable scent helps you fall asleep

During the Roman Empire, distinguished citizens added lavender to their bath water and used to carry a lavender bouquet in their clothes to ward off insects and emanate a soft and delicate aroma. Not surprisingly, it is one of the most commonly used medicinal plants in cosmetics and aromatherapy. It adds a fragrance to the air and repels moths. Placing its dried flowers in cloth sacks will add a light and pleasant, refreshing fragrance to your closet.

When should you use it?

Its balancing and sedative effect on the central nervous system reduces anxiety, nervous irritability, and stress. It is an effective treatment for insomnia because it promotes sleep, decreases motor activity, and lengthens the duration of sleep, so you get natural and restful sleep.

Furthermore, it is digestive, carminative, and antispasmodic, so it is great for facilitating and enhancing digestion, and eliminating annoying intestinal gas. Using its essential oil externally relaxes your muscles and relieves rheumatic pains of the joints and muscles. It is also antiseptic and healing, which helps treat infected wounds and burns, and alleviates the discomfort of insect bites.

Presentation

It is often found as dried and chopped flowers for tea (one teaspoon per cup of water every eight hours) and essential oil (one to four drops every eight hours). It can also be found in combination with other sedatives or digestive plants for preparing infusions.

Remedies

BY ITSELF
Relaxing and digestive infusion: place a teaspoon of lavender in a cup and add boiling water. After ten minutes, strain it and drink it after meals. Nothing relaxes your body and mind as much as taking a bath infused with a few drops of lavender essential oil.

COMBINED
Infusion to calm the nerves: you will get good results from brewing an herbal tea made by mixing equal parts lavender and other soothing plants such as linden or passionflower and drinking three cups a day. If instead you combine it with plants such as chamomile, pennyroyal, and anise, and drink it after meals, you will see great improvement in your digestion.

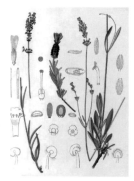

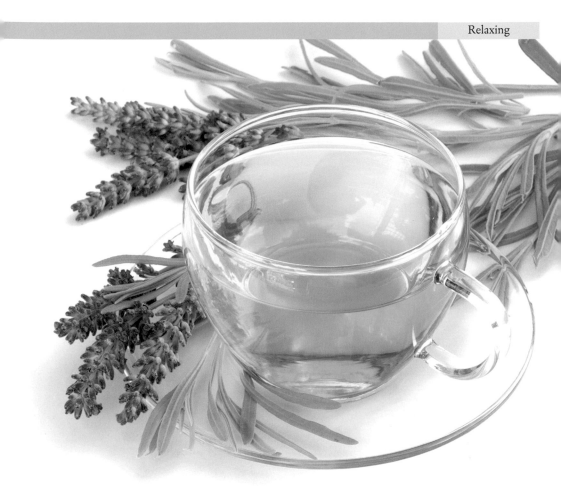

Precautions

It is contraindicated during pregnancy and lactation and for those suffering gastritis and peptic ulcer. As for the essential oil, be careful when administering it to young children, and do not use more than the recommended doses or for extended periods of time due to its potential neurotoxicity.

Description

It is a shrub that can grow up to 2 feet (60 centimeters) high. Its leaves are grayish green, narrow, and elongated, and its violet flowers are small and grouped in terminal spikes that are very aromatic.

Cultivation

It grows wild in chalky, dry, and sunny soil in southern Europe.

Harvesting

It blooms in summer. For therapeutic purposes, its inflorescences and leaves are harvested from July to August. It is dried in the shade, below 95°F (35°C), since at higher temperatures its essence gets altered and the plant's effectiveness is lost.

Composition

It has valuable essential oil content, as well as tannins, phenolic acids, flavonoids, triterpenes, and steroids.

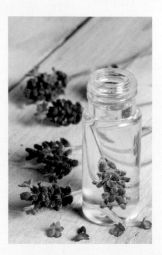

Hop

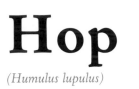

(Humulus lupulus)

Balances the mood

A traditional remedy for sleep is to rest on a pillow filled with its flower cones (strobili). Since antiquity, hop has been used as a tranquilizer. Since the Middle Ages, it has been used for brewing beer because it imparts a unique aroma and flavor along with preservative qualities.

When should you use it?

This plant's medicinal use is primarily centered around its sedative virtues. It is recommended for restlessness, nervous tension, and to prevent discomfort caused by anxiety. Its safety has been confirmed by its traditional use in beer, and it is very useful for getting a serene and restful sleep. It also prevents headaches stemming from body tension, as well as digestive disorders such as intestinal cramps and indigestion. As an infusion, hop is effective for stimulating appetite and improving digestive functions. It also has a slight estrogenic action.

Applied externally, this plant's vulnerary and antiseptic properties make it an effective remedy for acne, eczema, and dermatitis.

Presentation

You can find it on its own, dried and crushed for preparing infusions, but it is primarily found as a blend mixed with other sedative plants. You may also find it as capsules (doses are indicated by the manufacturer), liquid extract (⅛ teaspoon [0.5 milliliters] divided into 3 daily doses), and tincture (½ teaspoon [2.5 milliliters] divided into 3 daily doses). The last 2, when used to treat insomnia, can be taken as a single dose before bedtime.

Remedies

BY ITSELF

Relaxing infusion: place a teaspoon of hops in a cup and add boiling water. Let it steep for 10 to 15 minutes and strain. It can be sweetened with a little sugar or honey. Drink 3 cups a day, especially once before bedtime.

COMBINED

It can be used with other sedative plants such as valerian, linden flower, and lavender to improve and enhance sleep. For nervous indigestion, combine it with chamomile.

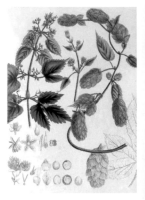

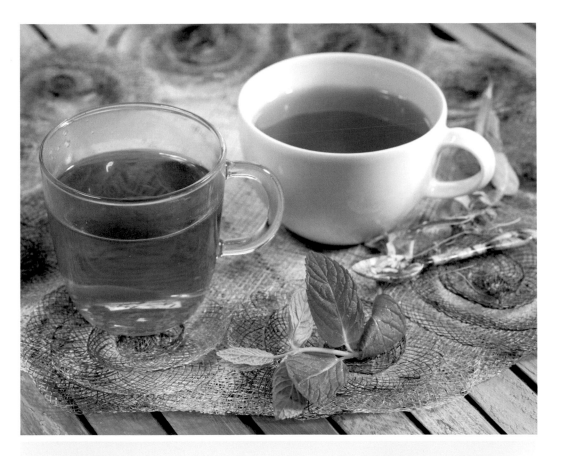

Precautions
Although it is a very safe medicinal plant and there are no adverse reactions to therapeutic doses, at high doses it may cause nausea and vomiting. It is contraindicated during pregnancy and lactation.

Description
It is a perennial climbing plant with twining stems that curl for support. The female flowers gather in inflorescences resembling cones, which are the strobili.

Cultivation
Native to the wet and cold regions of Europe, it grows wild in hedges, weeds, near forests, or along rivers.

Harvesting
The part that is used is the strobili (female inflorescences), which can be collected from late summer to fall. They are dried in the shade and stored in airtight containers, for one year at most.

Composition
Its main active ingredients are bitter floroglucinols, essential oil, phenolic acids, tannins, and flavonoids.

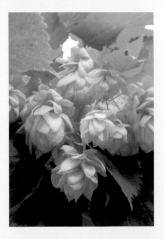

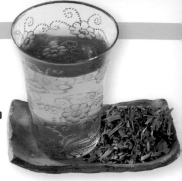

Passionflower

(Passiflora incarnata)

Great ally against stress

It is notable for its beautiful flower, which made European settlers in the New World name it after the passion of Christ. Later it was introduced into Europe for ornamental purposes, until the late 19th century, when its sedative properties became known.

When should you use it?

It is one of the best remedies to reduce nervousness and anxiety, and prevent insomnia. Its sedative effect calms the nerves and relaxes the muscles. It is recommended during stressful situations, such as personal or work-related problems, and to relieve pain associated to psychosomatic diseases. It also reduces nervous excitability associated with menopause and PMS. It is also especially useful for sleep disorders, because it is very effective at promoting sleep naturally, and it can be used without any problems in children and older adults to facilitate their sleep.

Its antispasmodic effect is very useful to prevent muscle spasms, intestinal spasms, and night cramps.

Presentation

It is most often found in the form of capsules or tablets alone or mixed with other sedative plants, with appropriate doses indicated by the manufacturer. It is also easy to find as dry and ground powder for tea (1 teaspoon per cup), in liquid extract (½ teaspoon [2 milliliters] every 8 hours), and tincture (¹⁄₁₆ teaspoon [0.52 milliliters] every 8 hours). You may see that it is a common ingredient in sedative syrups for both children and adults.

Remedies

BY ITSELF

Infusion to reduce anxiety: add a teaspoon of passionflower to a cup of boiling water. Let it steep for 10 minutes and strain. If you prefer, you can sweeten it with honey or sugar and drink up to 3 cups a day, every 8 hours.

COMBINED

Make tea by combining passionflower, lavender, hop, lemon balm, and valerian. Drink it to help you sleep, reduce stress and anxiety, or for intestinal spasms. It works very well in combination with other plants such as orange blossom, Saint John's wort, chamomile, and linden.

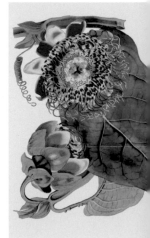

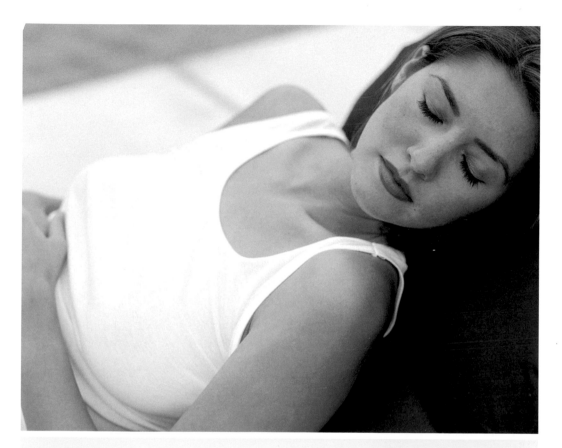

Precautions
The recommended dose is very safe but it is contraindicated during pregnancy and lactation. It can also enhance the effect of other sedative drugs, so do not take them together.

Description
It is a climbing plant known for its beautiful white flowers and double crown of purple filaments.

Cultivation
It is native to North America, and it grows spontaneously in dry and argillaceous soil that is especially rich in nutrients and where it is sunny.

Harvesting
The parts of the plant that are used are those found above ground consisting of stems, leaves, and flowers. It is gathered when in bloom between July and October. Then it is dried and stored in closed containers away from light and moisture.

Composition
Its chemical composition includes flavonoids, cyanogenic glycosides, phenolic acids, coumarins, steroids, essential oil, and trace amounts of alkaloids.

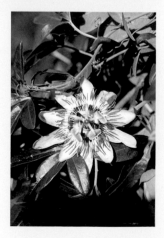

Linden flower

(Tilia cordata)

Calms and soothes coughing

Linden trees are somber and elegant, and seem to want to lead us toward a more calm and serene lifestyle. In central and northern European countries, they are a symbol of family unity. They also provide natural protection against the sun, because during the summer they can keep us cool, and in the winter they do not create much shade. Its use as a sedative dates back to the Renaissance, and today it is one of the most commonly used herbal remedies.

When should you use it?

Linden is prized as a sedative, so it is an effective and safe remedy to calm nervousness and anxiety. It can also be used for restful sleep if you suffer from insomnia, with the added advantage that the next morning you will not wake up feeling drowsy. Having no side effects, it is especially useful for anxious children who have trouble sleeping. Its antitussive, demulcent, and antispasmodic effect works in both children and adults to soothe coughing and cold symptoms and to sweat out a cold fever.

Popularly, it is also used as a diuretic, to relieve stomach discomfort, and slow digestion.

Applied externally, it protects the skin against the harsh effects of the wind, cold, or sun, and its emollient effect is recommended for eczema and skin irritations.

Presentation

You will find it most often prepared for infusion (1 teaspoon per cup) dried and cut, which you can buy by weight or in teabags with adequate dosages. It is as common to find it by itself as well in a blend with other, primarily sedative plants for treating colds and flu. It can also be in the form of capsules, liquid extract (½ teaspoon [2 milliliters] every 12 hours), and tincture (2 teaspoons [10 milliliters] every 12 hours).

Remedies

By Itself
Sedative infusion: boil briefly a teaspoon of dried flowers (about ½ teaspoon [2 grams]) per cup of water. Let it steep for 5 to 10 minutes and filter it. Drink it hot, up to 3 infusions per day. It calms the nerves and helps you fall asleep if you take it before going to bed.

Combined
Antitussive and expectorant infusion: mix equal parts linden, thyme, mullein, lungwort, and mallow. Take a teaspoon of this mixture and add it to a cup of boiling water, let it steep for 10 minutes, and strain. Drink 3 cups a day, which can be sweetened with sugar or honey.

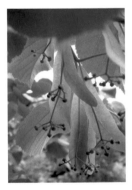

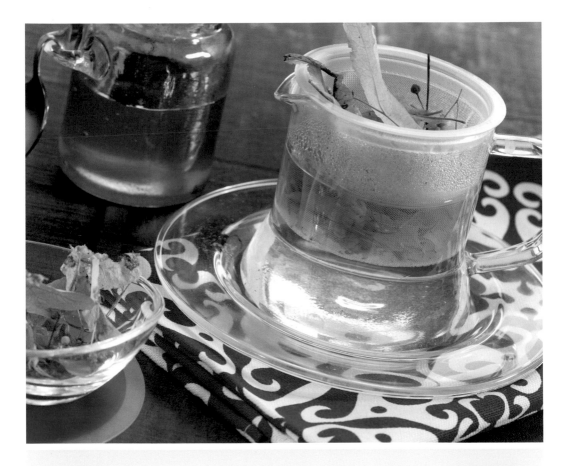

Precautions
It is not toxic so even infants can have it without any problems.

Description
It is an attractive deciduous tree with a long lifespan that grows up to 98 feet (30 meters) high. Its heart-shaped leaves, with serrated edges, are dark green on top and silvery green on the underside. Its fragrant flowers are greenish yellow and grown in inflorescences.

Cultivation
It grows spontaneously in mountain areas with cold and wet climate, such as beech, maple, and rowan forests. It is frequently grown in the Mediterranean region.

Harvesting
Its flowers and bracts are the parts that are used in herbal medicine. These are harvested in dry periods, when two-thirds of the plant is open. They are dried in a well-ventilated place and stored in tightly sealed containers away from light.

Composition
It contains mucilage, flavonoids, essential oil, tannins, and phenolic acids.

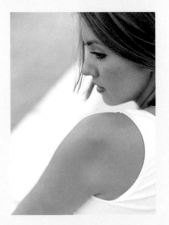

Valerian

(Valeriana officinalis)

Balances the nervous system

It was known back in ancient Greece, where it was used as a tranquilizer. Since then, it has been used for medicinal purposes, and today its known sedative effects are being researched in multiple studies.

When should you use it?

Valerian soothes the nerves, lowers blood pressure, relaxes the muscles, and is very effective for falling asleep and improving the quality of sleep, although it is not well known to which active substance these benefits can be attributed. It also has a markedly antispasmodic action, reinforcing its sedative effect, which makes it very useful for reducing anxiety and stress. It is also effective at preventing headaches, calming irritability associated with premenstrual syndrome and menopause, and easing painful abdominal spasms and intestinal gas.

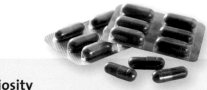

Curiosity

Take capsules and tablets with a glass of water, at least two hours before bedtime, because it sometimes has an adverse reaction of hyperexcitability that causes anxiety and insomnia.

Presentation

Because of its unpleasant taste and aroma, you will most commonly find it in capsules and tablets, either alone or combined with other sedative plants. The plant, dried and cut, can be bought by weight or in teabags. It is also available in liquid extract (¼ to 1 teaspoon [2 to 3 milliliters] 3 times a day) and tincture (⅛ to 1 teaspoon [1 to 3 milliliters] 3 times a day).

Remedies

BY ITSELF

Relaxing infusion: mix a teaspoon of valerian root to a cup of boiling water. Let it steep for 10 minutes and strain it. To hide its bad taste, sweeten with sugar or honey. To calm anxiety, drink up to three cups a day. For insomnia, drink a cup of tea at least an hour before going to sleep.

COMBINED

Infusion for sleeping: mix equal parts valerian, passionflower, and hawthorn. Add a teaspoon of this mixture to a cup of boiling water, let it steep for 10 minutes, strain it, and drink it hot, 1 hour before bedtime. It works especially well when insomnia is caused by anxiety or stress.

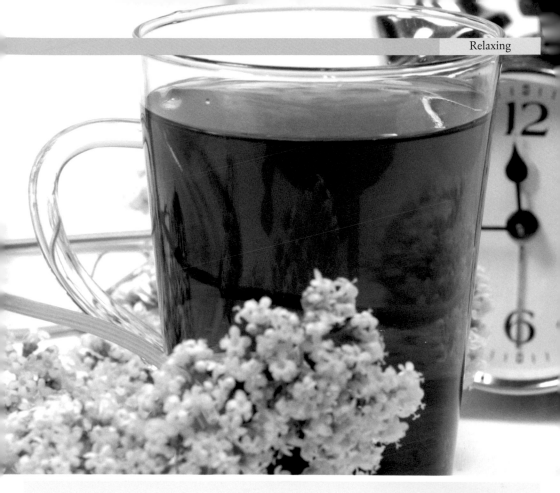

● **Precautions**
Although it is a fairly safe species, its use is not recommended for extended periods of time and it should be used with caution for those suffering from liver failure. On the other hand, its use is not recommended for pregnant or nursing women, or children under the age of 12, because although it is a widely used remedy, there are no studies to ensure its safety.

● **Description**
This plant grows 1.5 to 3 feet (50 to 100 centimeters) high, it is robust and unbranched. The upper leaves are shorter than the lower stalk, and its white or pink flowers grow in inflorescences. Its root has a very unpleasant odor when dry, but when it is fresh it does not smell at all.

● **Cultivation**
It grows in humid forests, river banks, and meadows throughout most of Europe.

● **Harvesting**
The usable parts of the plant lie underground (roots, rhizomes, and stolons) and are harvested in early autumn, then they are dried in a ventilated place and kept in closed containers away from light and moisture.

● **Composition**
Its main active ingredients are iridoid (valepotriates), essential oils, sesquiterpenes, lignans, phenolic acids, steroids, tannins, and traces of alkaloids.

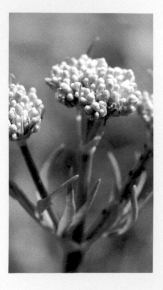

Verbena

(Verbena officinalis)

Against anxiety

Known as witchcraft herb, it has been traditionally and widely used in European magical tradition. The Greeks, Romans, and ancient Celts regarded it as a sacred plant that could protect them from all evil. Traditionally, it was harvested in summertime on the night of San Juan, when neither the sun nor the moon could be seen in the sky.

When should you use it?

It is recommended for anxiety, nervousness, and insomnia because it has an active sedative effect on the central nervous system. It is also used to relieve headaches associated with stress and menstruation, as well as for loss of appetite or listlessness caused by stress.

Moreover, this remedy can soothe the respiratory mucosa and prevent whooping cough. Its infusion, ingested as a drink and used for gargling, relieves angina and sore throat. It also stimulates appetite and the production of gastric juice, thereby improving poor digestion. It is a good diuretic to treat water retention and kidney disease.

Applied externally, it is an astringent remedy for healing minor wounds and burns.

Presentation

It is not a very common remedy in our country, but you might still find it on its own or as part of a mixed blend for making tea (one teaspoon per cup). It is also found in liquid extract (½ to ¾ teaspoon [2 to 4 milliliters] every 8 hours) and tincture (1 to 2 teaspoons [5 to 10 milliliters] every 8 hours).

Remedies

BY ITSELF

Relaxing infusion: add a teaspoon of verbena to a cup of boiling water. Let it steep for 5 to 10 minutes and strain. To calm the nerves, you only need to drink 1 cup a day.

COMBINED

Herbal tea to reduce stress and anxiety: mix equal parts verbena, passionflower, and oats. Add a spoonful of this mixture to a cup of boiling water and let it steep for 10 minutes. Then strain it and drink it hot. Drink 2 cups a day.

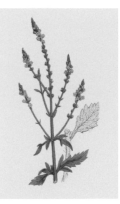

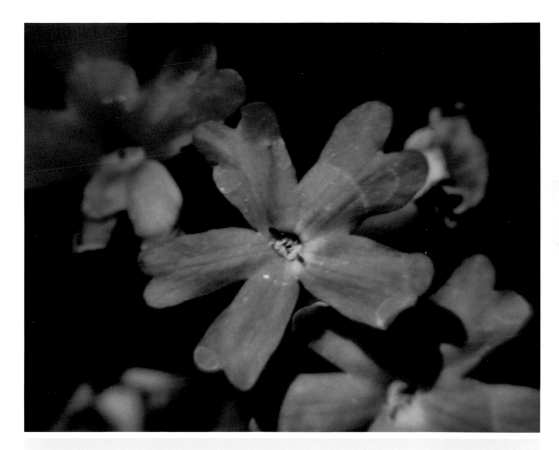

● Precautions

It has no side effects, but it is not recommended during pregnancy or lactation, and for small children. It should not be taken with sedatives or alcohol, as doing so would enhance its effect.

● Description

Inconspicuous herbaceous plant that grows up to 3 feet (1 meter) high. Its erect stems shoot out its lanceolate, hairy leaves. Its small violet flowers are grouped in spikes.

● Cultivation

It is a weed that has spread throughout the temperate zones of the earth.

● Harvesting

For therapeutic uses, its flowering tops are harvested when they begin to bloom (in summer) until the end of autumn. They are dried in the shade in a well-ventilated area, preferably with natural heat, and kept in closed containers away from moisture.

● Composition

It contains iridoid (verbenalina), flavonoids, and phenylpropane derivatives.

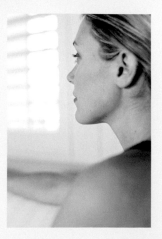

Damiana

(Turnera diffusa)

Tonic and aphrodisiac

This pleasantly aromatic flavor is used in Mexico as a substitute for tea. It also enjoys great fame as an aphrodisiac. In fact, the Mayas used this plant to increase their sexual potency and improve their sex lives. But traditionally, this plant has been widely used as a diuretic, laxative, and headache treatment.

When should you use it?

Damiana has toning and stimulating effects on the nervous system. It combats fatigue by providing energy and vigor without overstimulation or anxiety, unlike other stimulants. Its action is smooth and does not cause addiction. It is good for weakness or asthenia during seasons with little sunlight, symptoms of sadness, lack of interest, reduced sexual desire, and lack of concentration. It is also used as a supplement to treat impotence due to psychological issues. Its diuretic and antibacterial effect makes it a good remedy to treat cystitis and other urinary tract infections. By increasing urination, it helps prevent kidney stones. This plant also has a mild purgative effect, which works as a laxative when taken in excessive amounts.

Presentation

In Spain it is not very common, but it can still be found dried and ground, ready for making tea (one teaspoon per cup). It is also found in capsules or tablets, the dose indicated by the manufacturer, and as a tincture (½ to ¾ teaspoon [2 to 3 milliliters] 3 times a day).

Damiana is often more effective when combined with other herbs of similar or complementary activity.

Remedies

By ITSELF
Energizing infusion: prepare it by adding a teaspoon of dried leaves to a cup of boiling water. Let it steep for 10 to 15 minutes and strain. Drink up to 3 cups each day to help you stay in a good mood.

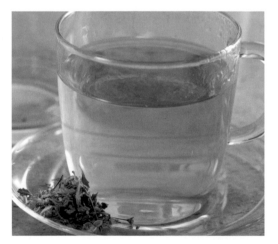

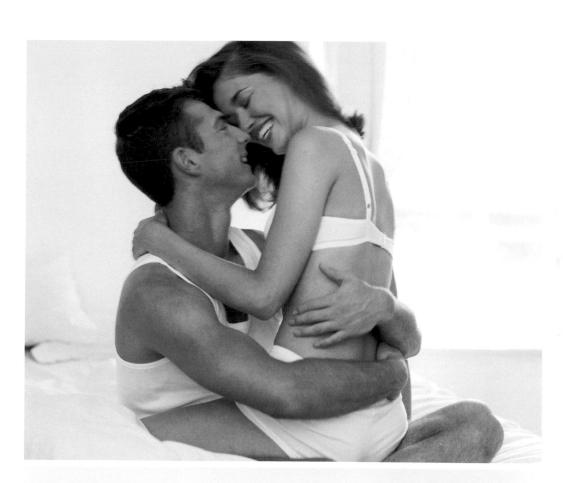

Precautions
At recommended doses there are no side effects, but it is contra-indicated during pregnancy and lactation, and for those suffering from hypertension, heart disease, anxiety, nervousness, and insomnia. It should not be taken with other stimulants.

Description
It is a shrub that can grow up to 6.5 feet (2 meters) high. Its small leaves have serrated edges and are lighter on the underside. Its blue or yellow flowers are small and bloom in late summer.

Cultivation
It grows in dry areas of the tropical American region; its shrubs grow at sea level and up at over 6,500 feet (2,000 meters) above sea level.

Harvesting
For medicinal use, its leaves are picked just when the plant is in full bloom. They are then sun-dried and stored in closed containers away from light and moisture.

Composition
It contains essential oil, tannins, simple phenols, and cyanogenic glycosides.

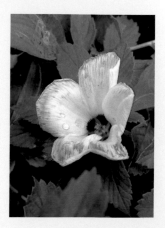

Spirulina

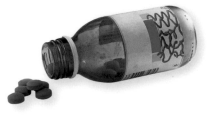

(Spirulina maxima)

Nutrient concentrate

Although spirulina is an algae that grows spontaneously in salty lakes in Mexico and the African continent, it is easy to grow. There are historical records where Spanish conquistadors suggest that the Aztecs harvested it and used it for food.

When should you use it?

It is used as a tonic because it is rich in nutrients. It helps to strengthen and restore the body after physical effort and nutritional deficiency due to unbalanced diets. It is also beneficial during recovery from convalescence and when you have low energy.

In addition, it is rich in chlorophyll, folic acid, iron, and vitamin B12, which promotes the production of red blood cells, and it has an anti-anemic effect.

It contains B vitamins and minerals like iron, magnesium, and zinc, making it a good resource to protect and enhance the health of skin, nails, and hair. It is rich in mucilage, so it is recommended for weight loss. It gives the sensation of "fullness," so it is good for reducing your appetite and keeping you from eating more than necessary. It works as a laxative for treating cases of chronic constipation. It also softens and reduces inflammation in the digestive mucosa, so it is helpful for gastritis and peptic ulcer.

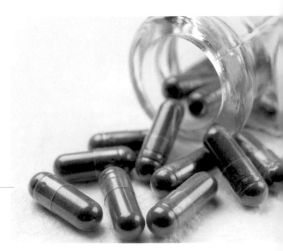

Presentation

Spirulina is easily found as capsules, tablets, or powders, so their indicated dosages will vary accordingly. In any case, it is best to consult with a specialist to obtain the right dosage amount.

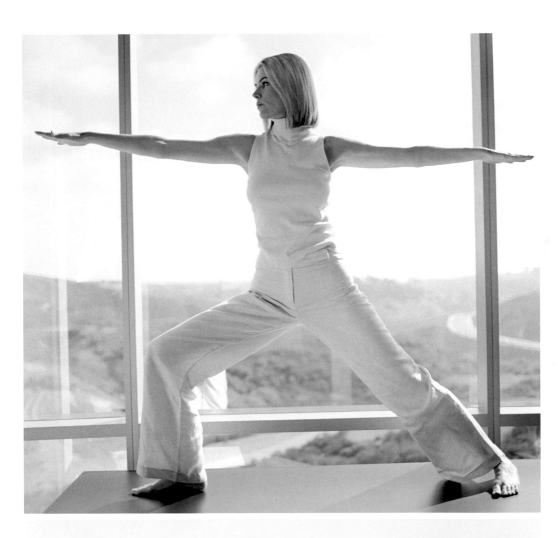

● **Precautions**
It is not toxic, but use it with caution during pregnancy and lactation.

● **Description**
It is a blue-green multicellular algae with a spiral thallus.

● **Cultivation**
It was discovered in Mexican lakes, but it grows and multiplies in natural alkaline waters. Today, it is grown in several countries.

● **Harvesting**
It is harvested throughout the year.

● **Composition**
It contains proteins and amino acids, mucilage, unsaturated fatty acids, vitamins, and minerals (especially iodine).

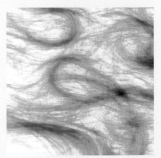

Guarana

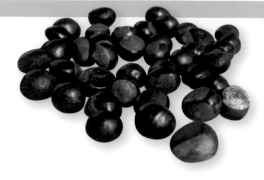

(Paullina cupana)

Helps restore vitality

The natives of Brazil have been using guarana since ancient times. They thought it was a magical fruit for curing intestinal diseases and regaining lost strength, quickly and safely. Even now, they claim that guarana powder can cure many diseases, but what is clear is that carbonated and energy drinks with guarana tone and stimulate the system for combating fatigue.

When should you use it?

It stimulates the central nervous system due to its content of caffeine and other stimulants, so it is effective at prolonging wakefulness and increasing your capacity for physical effort. As a general tonic and stimulant, it is a very useful remedy for physical fatigue, asthenia, tiredness, and bad mood. Furthermore, guarana is a diuretic and bronchodilator.

Its stimulating and toning properties seem to speed up the elimination of accumulated fat in the body. For this reason, and for its diuretic effect, it is very frequently used as a weight loss supplement and for getting rid of cellulite. On the other hand, weight loss diets often cause fatigue, so guarana can help restore both your physical and mental vitality.

Presentation

Guarana powder (¼ teaspoon [1 gram] per day) can be found as capsules, and the manufacturer will indicate its recommended dosage. It can also be found in drinkable ampoules and as part of other preparations mixed with other stimulant plants. Furthermore, in the field of cosmetics, it is very easy to find it as an ingredient in creams and gels against cellulite.

Do not exceed ¼ teaspoon (1 gram) of powder per day, although this amount can be spread out into three times a day, after meals, with the last dose taken in the afternoon, several hours before bedtime.

It is contraindicated for hypertension, cardiac arrhythmias, gastritis, peptic ulcer, epilepsy, hyperthyroidism, insomnia, during pregnancy and lactation, and for children under the age of 12. It is also important to note that it should not be combined with other stimulants (ginseng, coffee, mate, etc.). Moreover, given that it can cause insomnia and nervousness, is not advisable to take it at bedtime.

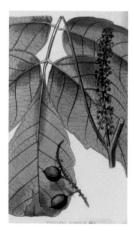

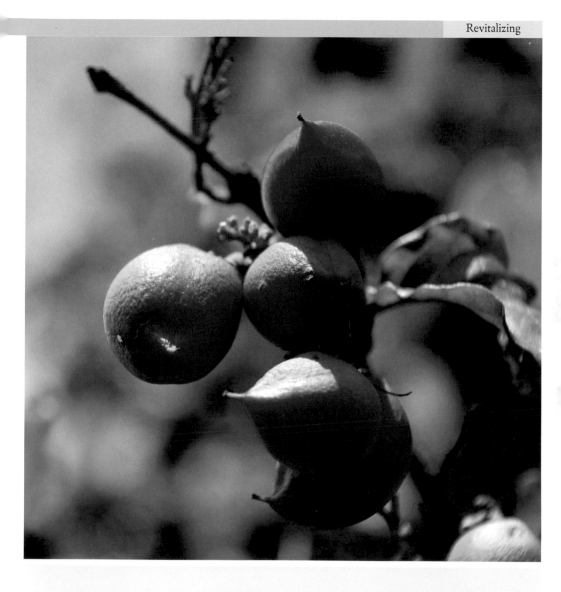

● Description
It is a shrub with peculiar small and round fruit, and it has a red or orange husk. When it ripens, it reveals its white flesh and black seeds, so that the fruits take on the appearance of a human eye.

● Cultivation
Native to the Amazon, it is grown in Brazil between Manaus and the Maués River.

● Harvesting
Traditionally, the fruits are gathered, the integument is removed from its seeds, then they are roasted and milled. The resulting powder is used for medicinal purposes.

● Composition
It contains a substance similar to caffeine (guaranine), other stimulants (caffeine, theobromine, and theophylline), tannins, and saponins.

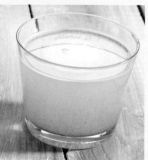

Saint John's wort

(Hypericum perforatum)

Anti-depressant and anti-anxiety remedy

Saint John's wort or Perforate St John's-wort is a medicinal plant that had a better reputation in classical antiquity. Known since Greek and Roman times, it is said that its name derives from the Greek *hyperikon* ("over an apparition"), a term which, according to some, refers to its ability to do away with evil spirits, something that was very important during the Middle Ages, when the plant was hung from the roofs of houses to prevent lightning and fire. It was also believed that to get these magical qualities, the plant had to be harvested in the morning of Saint John's day (summer solstice).

The word *perforatum* refers to the fact that Saint John's leaves are packed with secretory bags that are visible when backlit, like tiny holes, giving the plant a perforated appearance.

When should you use it?

Traditionally, Saint John's wort has been used as a remedy for healing wounds and urinary tract infections and for relieving nervous system disorders. However, it is now mainly regarded as an alternative remedy for treating mild and moderate depression, deterioration, lack of concentration, fatigue, and insomnia. Its effect is seen at least two weeks after starting treatment. In addition to its strong antidepressant effect, it is also an anti-anxiety remedy that can improve sleep and reduce stress and nervousness. Applied externally, it is effective for treating superficial wounds and minor burns, thanks to its antiseptic, anti-inflammatory, and healing action.

Presentation

Buying it in capsules and tablets is easier and practical. You can also find the tops, dried and ground, ready for making tea (1 teaspoon per cup); tincture (½ to ¾ teaspoon [2 to 4 milliliters] every 8 hours) and liquid extract (½ to ¾ teaspoon [2 to 4 milliliters] every 8 hours). There are drinkable ampoules where it is mixed with other plants.

Remedies

BY ITSELF

Antidepressant infusion: place a teaspoon of the plant in a cup and add boiling water. Let it steep for 10 minutes, strain, and if you like, sweeten it with a little honey or sugar. Drink up to 3 cups a day.

COMBINED

Herbal tea for depression with insomnia: mix equal parts Saint John's wort, heather, valerian, linden flower, and horehound. Add a teaspoon of this mixture to a cup of water and cook it over low heat for 2 minutes. Let it steep for 5 minutes, strain it, and drink it after dinner.

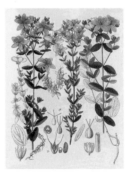

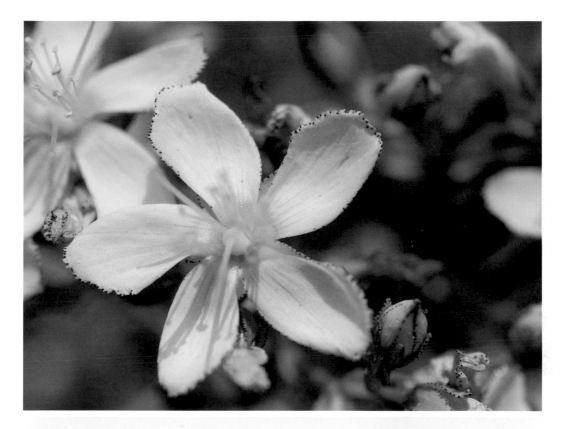

Precautions

It is contraindicated during pregnancy and lactation. If you are taking other medications, you need to consult with a specialist before using it. When taking Saint John's wort, avoid sun exposure since it is a photosensitizer.

Description

It is a perennial plant that grows 1 - to 2 feet (30 to 60 centimeters) high. Its stem is erect and its leaves have numerous translucent dots that look like holes in a raggedy piece of cloth. Its yellow flowers have five petals.

Cultivation

It grows all around the world, in pastures, lawns, roadsides, and open woodlands.

Harvesting

For medicinal purposes, its flowering tops are harvested from June to August. They have to be dried immediately in the shade and then placed in opaque glass bottles that are sealed tightly and kept in a cool, dry place.

Composition

Its many active ingredients include flavonoids, xanthones, phenolic acids, tannins, triterpenes, carotenoids, steroids, and essential oil.

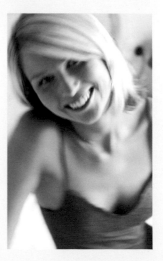

Kola nut

(Cola nitida)

Prevents fatigue

Historically, in Africa they have chewed kola seeds to increase mental alertness and fight fatigue. Now, fresh kola plays an important role in tropical societies for its ability to prevent fatigue, and as an important source of economic wealth, since a lot of its production line is intended for manufacturing nonalcoholic soft drinks.

When should you use it?

It is a powerful long-acting tonic that works as a physical and intellectual stimulant to prevent fatigue. It increases attention, intellectual speed, and brainstorming. It is useful during convalescence, in situations of prolonged fatigue, and to increase athletic performance. It is also used to reduce weakness and anxiety.

It has a strong diuretic effect that helps to prevent fluid retention. It is also an effective remedy to relieve headaches.

Presentation

You can find the whole nut (take ½ to 1 teaspoon [2 to 6 grams] per day), dry (0.2 to 0.7 grams per day), in liquid extract (up to 30 drops twice a day), and in capsules (1 or 2, twice per day).

Remedies

BY ITSELF

The whole nut can be slowly chewed, or it can be prepared as an infusion to drink, preferably after eating.

Another nice way to enjoy it is by making kola wine. Marinate for a few days 3 tablespoons (50 grams) of powdered seeds in 1 cup (250 grams) of alcohol that is suitable for human consumption. Then add 3 cups (700 milliliters) of wine and leave it marinating for 3 months. Filter it and drink 3 cups a day as a general tonic.

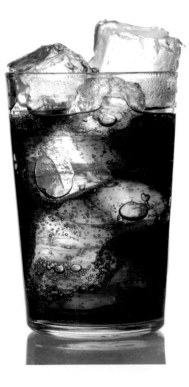

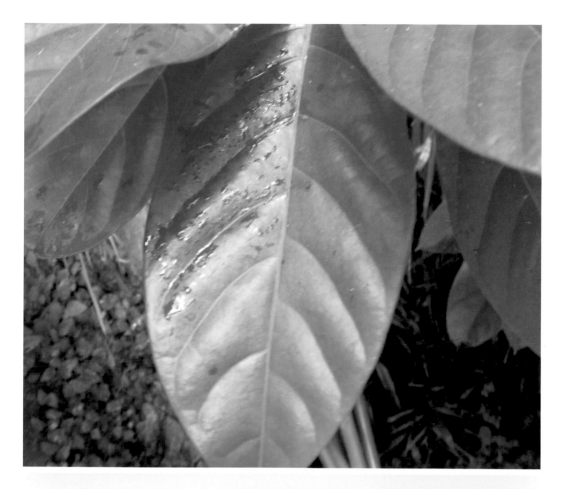

● **Precautions**
It is contraindicated for those suffering from insomnia, anxiety, and nervousness. It should not be used during pregnancy and lactation, for children under the age of twelve, or those under-going treatment for peptic ulcer, hypertension, arrhythmia, or hyperthyroidism. It should not be taken with other stimulants or when you are treated with digitalis.

● **Description**
It is a large tree that is characterized by flowers that have no corolla and grow grouped in small clusters in the leaf axils.

● **Cultivation**
It is native to tropical Africa and other tropical countries.

● **Harvesting**
Seeds without their integument are used.

● **Composition**
It contains xanthine bases such as caffeine, theophylline, and theobro-mine, as well as tannins, carbo-hydrates, lipids, and mineral salts.

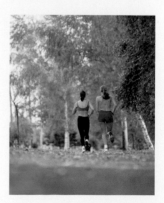

Green tea

(Camellia sinensis)

A stimulating antioxidant drink

Green tea is one of the oldest beverages in the world, which according to Chinese legend, was discovered accidentally by an emperor four thousand years ago. Since then, green tea continues to be a preferred beverage in Asian countries (China, Japan, and India), where it has been used in traditional medicines. Currently, it is consumed by more than two thirds of the world's population and is the second most consumed beverage after water.

When should you use it?

Tea is a very popular infusion because of its stimulating effect on the central nervous system. It stimulates your metabolism and increases wakefulness. These properties make it effective for physical and mental exhaustion and asthenia. It also tones your muscles, improves breathing, and has a bronchodilator effect that is good for treating bronchitis and asthma. It also increases gastric juices, improves digestion, and is an effective diuretic to prevent fluid retention.

It is recommended for treating obesity because it facilitates the elimination of fluids, and it accelerates the elimination of fat, while its stimulating effect is good for combating weakness that is often associated with low-calorie diets. It also lowers blood cholesterol levels and has great antioxidant and antibiotic action. For external use, green tea reduces localized accumulations of fat (cellulite) as an ingredient in creams and gels, which need to be applied every day to be effective.

Presentation

It is available as a tea (1 teaspoon per cup) in capsules filled with dry leaves, liquid extract (½ teaspoon [2.5 milliliters] every 8 hours), in drops, and ampoules. Green tea is part of numerous oral medications for weight loss and for external application against cellulite in the form of gels or creams.

Remedies

BY ITSELF

Stimulating infusion: place a teaspoon of green tea in a cup of boiling water. Let it steep for 2 minutes and strain. If you want to use as a diuretic, let it steep for 5 minutes. Either way, drink 3 cups a day.

COMBINED

Invigorating infusion: mix equal parts green tea, lemon balm, and rosehips. Add a teaspoon of this mixture to a cup of boiling water and let it steep for 10 minutes. Strain it and drink a cup after meals. It is great for restoring your energy.

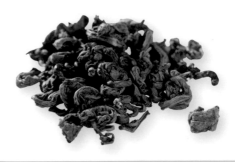

Antioxidant effect

Green tea's high content of catechins offer a valuable antioxidant and metabolic activator. In fact, recent research determined that green tea contains the most potent antioxidant known to date (epigallocatechin gallate). This makes it very effective in preventing premature aging. Experts have not yet agreed about the best dose, but it is known that in China and Japan, where there are lower rates of degenerative diseases, people drink three to four cups a day.

● Precautions

Green tea should not be used for hypertension, cardiac arrhythmias, gastritis, peptic ulcer, epilepsy, hyperthyroidism, anxiety, insomnia, during pregnancy and lactation, and for children under the age of 12. It hinders the absorption of dietary iron, so it should not be used when suffering from anemia. If you abuse it, it can cause insomnia and anxiety.

● Description

It is a perennial, very branched shrub that grows to 33 feet (10 meters) high.

● Cultivation

It is native to northern India and southern China. It multiplies through seeds and grows in moist soils in a warm climate.

● Harvesting

Its leaves are harvested when the plant is 3 years old, and they are usually harvested 3 times a year.

● Composition

It contains xanthine bases such as caffeine, theophylline, and theobromine, as well as tannins, flavonoids, phenolic acids, organic acids, saponins, and essential oil.

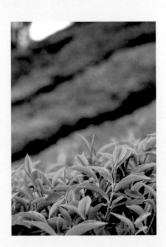

Horseweed

(Erigeron canadensis)

Effective anti-rheumatic

Native people of North America have been using it since ancient times for its medicinal properties. Traditionally, they used it to stop heavy menstrual periods.

When should you use it?

This is a plant with diuretic and anti-inflammatory properties, so it is recommended for treating rheumatism and osteoarthritis because it alleviates inflammatory joint pain effectively. Besides its anti-rheumatic properties, it prevents gout and its diuretic effect helps the absorption of edema (fluid retention).

Presentation

You can find the plant, dried and crushed, ready for making tea (2 teaspoons per cup) or decoctions, and as liquid extract (½ to ¼ teaspoon [1 to 2.5 milliliters] every 8 hours). However, it is common to use it in capsule with the ground and powder horseweed; the recommended dose is indicated by the manufacturer.

Remedies

BY ITSELF

Infusion for rheumatic pain: place 1 tablespoon of dried plant into a cup of boiling water. Let it steep for 10 minutes and strain. To relieve joint pain, drink up to 3 cups a day, after meals.

COMBINED

When combined with devil's claw and black currant it increases its potency to relieve rheumatic pains.

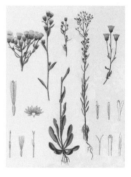

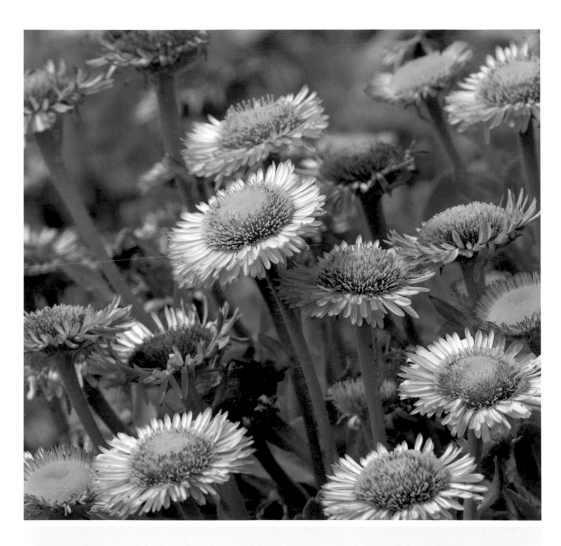

● **Precautions**
It is contraindicated for pregnant and nursing women and children.

● **Description**
This plant grows up to 3 feet (1 meter) high. It presents a thin and fusiform rhizome with a greenish erect stem. The leaves are alternate, stalked, and lanceolate. Small flower heads come together in clusters.

● **Cultivation**
It is native to North America.

● **Harvesting**
The flowering tops of the plant are used for medicinal purposes.

● **Composition**
It contains essential oils, tannins, and polyyne.

Ash

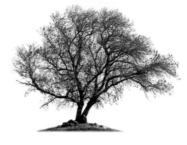

(Fraxinus excelsior)

Soothes joint pain

In Norse mythology, a large ash tree holds the world with its branches in the sky, its trunk on the ground, and its roots in the sea. In fact, its wood is highly valued for making boats, oars, even tool handles because of its water resistance, flexibility, and durability. However, ash not only has good wood, but its bark and leaves also have valuable medicinal properties.

When should you use it?

Traditionally, it has been used against rheumatic pain in the muscles and joints. It has been shown to have anti-inflammatory and diuretic effect. This facilitates the excretion of substances such as urea and urate. It is still used very effectively as a natural remedy against rheumatism, gout, and other painful inflammation. By increasing urinary excretion, it can prevent edema (fluid retention) and kidney stones. Also, thanks to its mucilage and mannitol content, it is a plant that has a mild laxative effect that relieves constipation, twenty-four hours after being administered.

Presentation

Most often, it is found in capsules with powdered plant (the dose is indicated by the manufacturer), but it is also possible to acquire the plant dry and chopped to prepare decoctions (½ to 2 tablespoons [10 to 30 grams] per 1 quart (1 liter) of water. Drink one or two cups a day.), in liquid extract (⅛ to ¼ teaspoon [0.5 to 1.5 milliliters] every 8 hours), and tinctures (½ to 1 teaspoon [2.5 to 5 milliliters] every 8 hours).

Remedies

BY ITSELF

Decoction for gout: boil 1 or 2 tablespoons of ash in a cup of water for a few minutes. Let it steep for 15 minutes and strain. Drink 3 cups a day, preferably after meals.

COMBINED

Infusion to relieve rheumatic pain: mix equal parts ash, black currant, nettle, meadowsweet, and Java tea. Add 1 tablespoon of this mixture to a cup of boiling water, let it steep for 10 minutes, and strain. Drink 1 cup every 8 hours. It relieves rheumatic pain associated with gout.

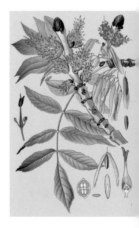

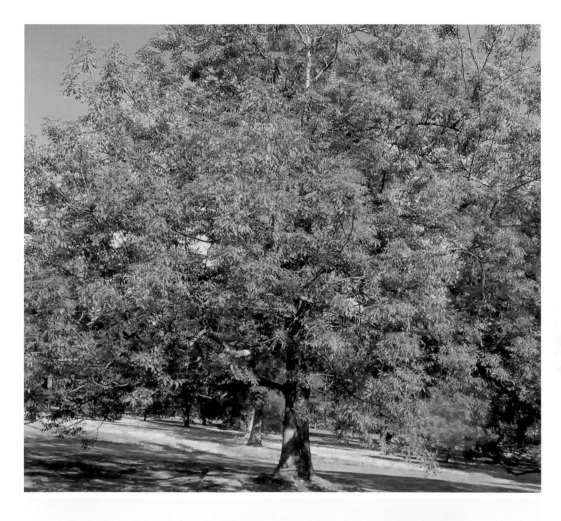

● Precautions
It is contraindicated if you suffer any type of intestinal obstruction, during pregnancy and lactation, and for young children. For kidney or heart failure, consult with a specialist before using it.

● Description
It is a large tree with smooth gray bark. Its leaves are oval and serrated, and its flowers are very inconspicuous.

● Cultivation
It is native to Europe and grows in forests, damp locations near the Atlantic, and along riverbanks.

● Harvesting
Its leaves and bark are used.

● Composition
It contains flavonoids, coumarins, organic acids, inositol, mucilage, phenolic acids, iridoids, and abundant mannitol.

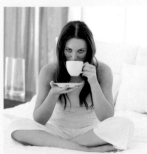

Black currant

(Ribes nigrum)

Diuretic and anti-inflammatory

Originally from northern Europe, it is well known for its delicious black fruits. However, in herbal medicine it is more appreciated for the medicinal virtues of its leaves, which are diuretic and anti-inflammatory. Among other uses, traditionally it is used to relieve pain and inflammation caused by insect bites.

When should you use it?

Black currant leaves have an important anti-inflammatory and anti-rheumatic action on rheumatism in general, without the disadvantages often presented by regular allopathic medicine. Its anti-inflammatory effect, related to its potent diuretic ability to eliminate waste substances such as urea and uric acid, also helps in the treatment of gout and to increase diuresis in genitourinary disorders such as cystitis. It is also a good weight-loss supplement to prevent fluid retention.

Moreover, this plant has an antispasmodic effect that can calm whooping cough and works as a powerful astringent to stop diarrhea. Its fruit has antioxidant vasoprotective and venotonic activity. Black currants effectively increase capillary resistance and decrease the permeability of the vein walls, giving very good results in the prevention of varicose veins and hemorrhoids. It has been used successfully for retinal microcirculation and to improve visual acuity, so it is recommended for retinitis pigmentosa or loss of night vision.

Presentation

You will most easily find its dried and chopped leaves (in troches), ready for making infusions (½ to 1 teaspoon [2 to 4 grams] per cup of water). It can also be used in capsules (the dosage recommended by the manufacturer) and syrup (1 teaspoon to 1 tablespoon [5 to 10 milliliters] every 8 hours). It is also included as a diuretic and anti-inflammatory plant in various mixtures for infusion.

Its fruits can be eaten fresh or in a juice.

Remedies

BY ITSELF

Diuretic infusion: place 2 to 3 teaspoons of dried leaves in a cup of boiling water. Let it steep for 10 minutes and strain. Drink 1 cup several times a day to increase diuresis and relieve rheumatic pain.

COMBINED

Diuretic infusion for joint discomfort: mix equal parts dandelion, black currant, and devil's claw. Place 1 or 2 tablespoons of this mixture in a cup and add boiling water. Let it steep for 10 minutes and strain. Drink up to 3 cups a day, after meals.

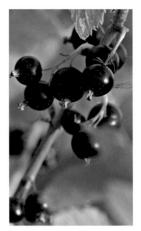

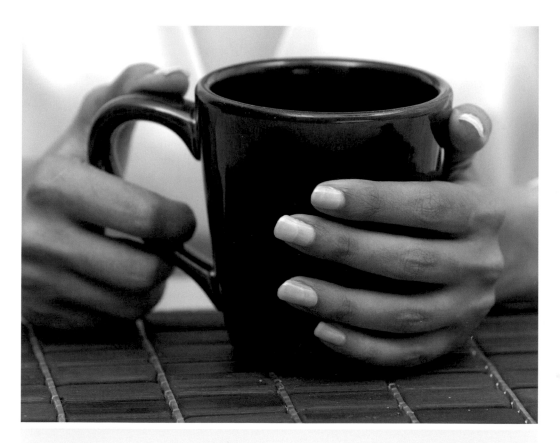

Precautions
The use of black currant leaves is contraindicated for pregnant women, nursing women, and young children. Persons suffering from renal failure, heart problems, or high blood pressure should consult with a specialist before using.

Description
It is an evergreen shrub that grows to 6.5 feet (2 meters) high. Its branches are hard and its leaves are alternate, stalked, with serrated edges and many resinous glands on the underside. Its flowers grow in dense clusters and its fruits are dark berries.

Cultivation
It grows spontaneously in central and eastern Europe and in temperate zones.

Harvesting
Its leaves and fruits are harvested in July and August. Its leaves are dried in the shade, and they are stored in pieces inside tightly closed glass containers, away from light.

Composition
Its leaves contain essential oils, flavonoids, catechic tannins, and organic acids. Its fruits contain flavonoids, anthocyanins, phenolic acids, organic acids, vitamin C, and minerals.

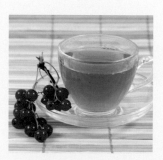

Devil's claw

(Harpagophytum procumbens)

Natural alternative for arthritis and osteoarthritis

Pain, stiffness, and loss of mobility are typical symptoms of rheumatic diseases, which are very common in people over sixty-five. Despite their high incidence, there is little effective treatment to alleviate the pain they cause. This medicinal plant is a good natural alternative for treating these ailments, in addition to allopathic treatments, helping to stop the inflammatory process and lessen pain with fewer side effects.

When should you use it?

It has analgesic, anti-inflammatory, and anti-arthritic properties. Whether used internally or externally, it is a particularly effective remedy for improving chronic inflammation and pain caused by rheumatic diseases such as arthritis and osteoarthritis. It also soothes dorsal, lumbar, and cervical pain and tendinitis. It can substitute or supplement synthetic anti-inflammatory medications that cause significant adverse side effects during prolonged treatment. Also, this remedy stimulates appetite and significantly improves indigestion because it stimulates the production and excretion of bile into the intestine, thereby helping to digest fats. As if this were not enough, it helps reduce cholesterol in the blood, and it has a mild laxative action.

Presentation

It is very common to find it as capsules and tablets because it has a very bitter taste, so this is the most practical way to ingest it. However, it is also quite common to use its dry root for preparing decoctions and as liquid extract (¼ teaspoon [1.5 milliliters] every 8 hours). You may also find it as an ingredient of anti-rheumatic tea blends.

Remedies

BY ITSELF

Anti-rheumatic maceration: place 2 teaspoons (4.5 grams) of the root of devil's claw in a container with 1 ¼ cup (300 milliliters) of water, and let it sit at room temperature for 8 hours. Then filter it and drink it throughout the day in 3 doses.

COMBINED

To reinforce its anti-rheumatic effect, combine it with white willow and Java tea. For example, you could prepare a very effective herbal tea to relieve symptoms of arthritis and gout by mixing 1 part white willow, 1 part devil's claw, and 2 parts Java tea. Place a teaspoon of this mixture into a cup of boiling water and let it steep for 10 minutes. Strain it and sweeten it with honey. Drink up to 3 cups a day, after meals.

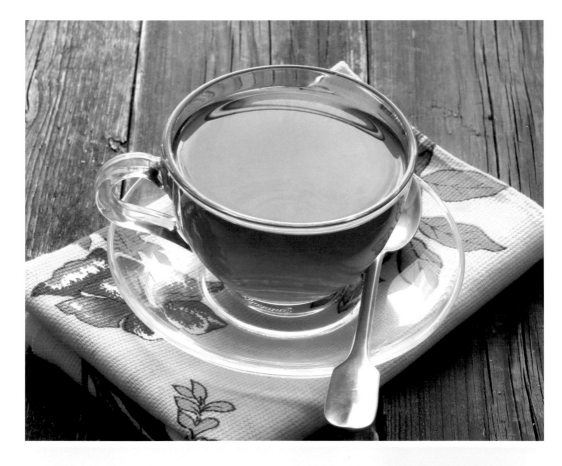

Precautions
It is contraindicated for persons suffering from peptic ulcer, gastritis, and biliary obstruction. Its use is not recommended during pregnancy and lactation and for small children.

Description
It is a creeping plant that draws attention for its secluded purple flowers. Its leaves are fleshy and hard, and its fruit, which lies at ground level, is thorny and woody. Its taproot is very long, and its lateral roots have a very bitter taste.

Cultivation
Native to southern Africa, it grows in sandy and argillaceous soil.

Harvesting
Its lateral roots are used. They are harvested by specially trained individuals, and once dried, they are crushed into small pieces. They are stored in tightly closed glass containers, away from light and moisture.

Composition
It contains iridoids, flavonoids, phenolic acids, triterpenes, and steroids.

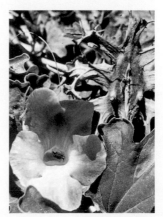

White willow

(Salix alba)

Effective weapon against pain

This plant has been used throughout the centuries in China, ancient Greece, and medieval Europe. Even Native Americans used it against headaches, fever, and muscle aches. In 1882, salicin was extracted from it, a substance that was soon purified into salicylic acid. This active ingredient is effective for pain and fever, but it is also sufficiently irritating to eliminate warts, so it was later changed (this time from meadowsweet) to create acetylsalicylic acid, the active ingredient in aspirin.

When should you use it?

Salicin has antipyretic, analgesic, anti-rheumatic, and antiseptic properties. It is an excellent natural remedy against mild febrile illness, such as colds or influenza, headaches, and inflammation.

It is also effective against rheumatic pain in muscles and joints, back pain, and tendinitis.

As interest in natural medicine increases, white willow has begun to be regarded as an alternative to aspirin.

Presentation

Willow bark has anti-rheumatic actions. It is also available mixed with devil's claw root in capsules and tablets. You will often find it as an ingredient in mixtures for infusion to treat colds and flu.

You can find it dry and chopped to make decoctions (2 teaspoons per cup), as liquid extract (¼ to ½ teaspoon [1 to 2 milliliters] every 8 hours), as a tincture (1 to 2 teaspoons [5 to 8 milliliters] every 8 hours), and in capsules with the proper dosage recommended by the manufacturer.

Remedies

BY ITSELF

Analgesic decoction: place 1 or 2 teaspoons of white willow in a cup of water and boil it for a few minutes. Let it steep for 5 minutes and filter it. Drink up to 4 cups, preferably after meals.

COMBINED

Decoction for pain: mix 1 part meadowsweet flower, 1 part elderflower, and 2 parts white willow bark. Place 2 teaspoons of this mixture in a cup of water and boil it for a few minutes. Let it steep for 15 minutes and strain it. Drink 2 cups a day, after meals.

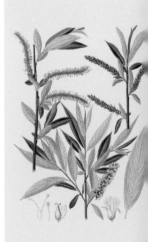

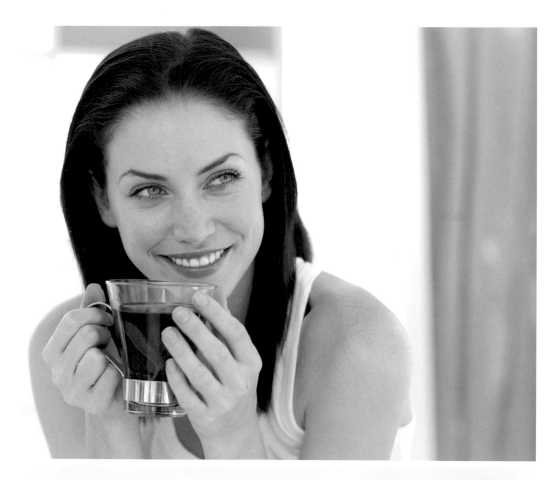

Precautions
Do not use if you are allergic to salicylates or if you are suffering from gastritis, peptic ulcer, asthma, or coagulation disorders. Do not administer to children younger than 16. Do not use during pregnancy or lactation.

Description
It is a deciduous tree that grows to 65 feet (20 meters) high. Its leaves have a serrated edge and are silvery gray. Its green bark is smooth in young trees and cracked in older trees.

Cultivation
It grows in warm and humid areas, and it cannot stand extreme temperatures.

Harvesting
Its cortex is used after it has been extracted from the branches that are 2 to 3 years old. It is dried separately from the woody part for several days in the shade, and it is stored in tightly closed containers, away from light and moisture.

Composition
It contains simple phenols (salicin, most importantly), tannins, and flavonoids.

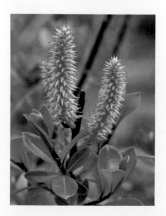

Meadowsweet

(Filipendula ulmaria)

Ally against rheumatism

Also known as "queen of the meadow," this beautiful plant has been used since the sixteenth century to soothe rheumatic pains. Just as with willow, the plant contains salicylates with antipyretic properties (fever reducers) that gave us the famous aspirin. In fact, the name "aspirin" comes from the Latin word Spiraea ulmaria.

When should you use it?

When some of its active ingredients are metabolized, they become salicylic derivatives with known anti-inflammatory, antipyretic, and analgesic properties. It also has a marked diuretic effect to help excretion of uric acid and urea. Therefore, this remedy is primarily used to treat muscle and joint rheumatism, and gout. It is also effective as treatment for influenza and febrile conditions, to prevent edema (fluid retention), and to prevent kidney stones. It also has some anticoagulant effect that contributes to the prevention of thromboembolism, so use it carefully if you are being treated with anticoagulants.

Presentation

It is most commonly available with other plants, in preparations (mixtures for infusion, capsules and tablets) to be used as anti-rheumatic remedies. It can be purchased on its own, dried and chopped to make tea (1 teaspoon per cup), as liquid extract (½ to ¾ teaspoon [2 to 3 milliliters] every 8 hours), and tinctures (½ to ¾ teaspoon [2 to 4 milliliters] every 24 hours).

Remedies

By itself

Anti-rheumatic infusion: add a teaspoon of dried flower tops to a cup of boiling water and let it steep for 10 minutes. Strain it and drink it after meals.

Decoction for external use: add ¼ cup (25 grams) of meadowsweet to 1 quart (1 liter) of water and boil it for 15 minutes. Strain it and use it to wash affected areas (no more than 10 minutes) to relieve both muscle and joint rheumatism.

Combined

For treating rheumatism, it gives very good results when combined with devil's claw, black currant, and willow bark.

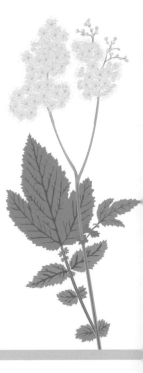

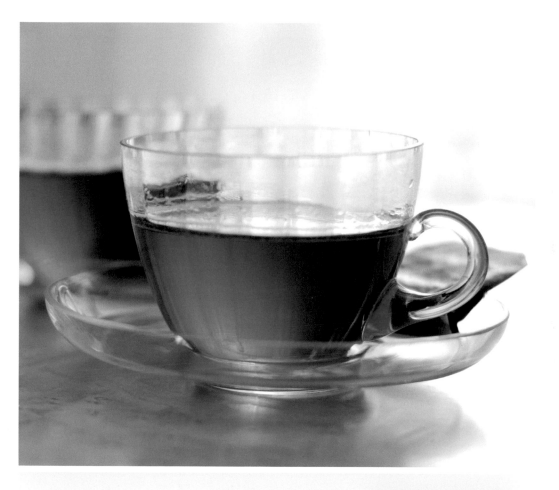

Precautions
It is contraindicated for persons allergic to salicylates, those suffering from peptic ulcer or gastritis, during pregnancy and lactation, and for young children. If you have asthma or bleeding disorders, you should consult with a specialist before using it.

Description
Herbaceous plant that can grow to 6.5 feet (2 meters) high. Its leaves are alternate and stalked, with jagged edges. Its small white flowers are clustered together in cymes.

Cultivation
It is native to Europe and grows spontaneously in moist meadows and near waterways.

Harvesting
Its flowering tops are harvested in summer, when its flowers have not completely opened. They are dried as soon as possible in the shade.

Composition
It contains essential oil, phenolic acids, flavonoids, anthocyanins, and tannins.

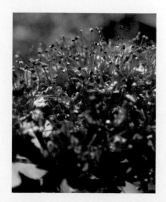

Eucalyptus

(Eucalyptus globulus)

A salve for the lungs

Native to Australia, this is one of the world's tallest trees. It was introduced in Europe in the late nineteenth century in order to drain swamps because as eucalyptus trees grow quickly, they absorb large amounts of water, but they acidify the soil and prevent other plants from growing around them.

When should you use it?

Whether fresh or dry, its leaves have expectorant, mucolytic, antispasmodic, antiseptic, and slightly antipyretic properties, so it is an excellent remedy for all respiratory diseases, especially colds, pharyngitis, and bronchitis. Its antiseptic effect is attributed to its essential oil, and although it mainly acts on the respiratory tract, it also has an effect on the urogenital tract, so it is also sometimes used to treat cystitis.

Topically, it also works well to relieve muscle and joint pain and heal wounds, and for gargling to mitigate pain in the mouth and throat.

Presentation

There are numerous eucalyptus preparations. Among the most common, there are infusions (by weight and in teabags), inhalations, tinctures (2 tablespoons [10 to 12 milliliters] every 12 hours), elixirs and syrups, liquid extract (½ - ¾ teaspoon [2 to 3 milliliters] every 12 hours), and essential oil (0.3 to 0.6 grams per 24 hours). It can also be taken as capsules made from its leaves. Eucalyptus essential oil is an ingredient in ointments and liniments, mouthwashes, inhalers to relieve nasal congestion, and medication for pain in the gums, mouth, and throat.

Remedies

BY ITSELF

Expectorant tea: pour a cup of boiling water over 1 teaspoon of dried leaves. Cover it and let it steep for about 10 minutes. Strain it and sweeten it with honey or sugar, if you like. Drink up to 3 cups a day, hot and freshly prepared.

COMBINED

Pectoral tea: mix equal parts eucalyptus, mullein, thyme, and greater plantain. Place a teaspoon of this mixture in a cup and add boiling water. Let it sit covered for 10 minutes and strain. Drink 1 hot cup every 8 hours to relieve cold symptoms.

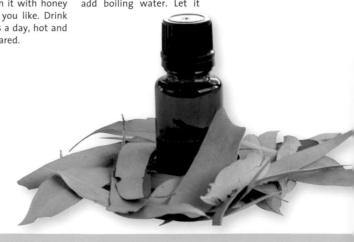

Eucalyptus vapor

Eucalyptus vapor is the best way to get all the properties of eucalyptus; in fact, it is the most widely used expectorant remedy. To make it, boil just enough eucalyptus leaves in water and inhale its vapor for 10 or 15 minutes. This remedy is a very effective nose decongestant and helps relieve coughing.

Precautions
It is contraindicated for persons suffering from peptic ulcer or gastritis, and during pregnancy and lactation. If you are suffering from liver failure, consult with a specialist before using. Its essential oil should be carefully administered to small children, without exceeding the recommended dosage. It should not be used in high doses or for extended periods of time due to its possible toxicity.

Description
It is a tall tree; in Europe some specimens grow to 98 feet (30 meters) high, but in Australia and America it is not uncommon to find some that grow to 328 feet (100 meters). Its trunk is smooth and light-colored, and its perennial leaves are lanceolate.

Cultivation
It is cultivated and naturalized in temperate regions of Europe and America. It prefers moist and marshy lands and does not support intense cold.

Harvesting
Leaves from adult branches are harvested throughout the year.

Composition
The most important element of its composition is its essential oil. It also contains other active ingredients such as flavonoids, triterpenes, tannins, and phenolic acids.

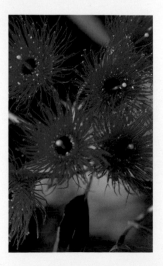

Mullein

(Verbascum thapsus)

Soothes and calms coughing

The pectoral virtues of this plant that smells like honey were known in Classical Greece. In Rome, the yellow pigments of flowers were used to lighten hair. Its velvety leaves have been used as dressings for wounds, and its stems were dried and covered with fat to be used as candlewicks.

When should you use it?

It has expectorant, cough suppressant, demulcent, antispasmodic, and sudorific properties, so it is especially suitable for treating conditions that cause irritation of the respiratory mucosa such as dry cough, pharyngitis, laryngitis, colds, bronchitis, and asthma. This plant calms coughing, softens and moisturizes the respiratory mucosa, and clears out the chest and lungs.

Its high content of mucilage helps regulate intestinal functions and eliminate constipation. Used externally, it has emollient properties (softens and moisturizes skin tissue), so it is an effective remedy for frostbite, skin irritations, stings, and hemorrhoids.

Presentation

It is not too widespread in our country, however, it is most commonly available dried and cut, sold by weight or in teabags for making infusions (1 teaspoon per cup), either alone or mixed with other ingredients for treating respiratory conditions. It can also be purchased in capsules, which is very convenient and safe since its dosage is already indicated by the manufacturer (½ tablespoon (7.5 - 10 ml) every 12 hours), and liquid extract (¼ teaspoon [1.5 to 2 milliliters] every 12 hours).

Remedies

BY ITSELF

Anti-cold infusion: place a teaspoon of mullein in a cup and add boiling water. Let it steep for 10 minutes and strain. It can be sweetened with honey or sugar. Drink 1 cup every 12 hours while it is still hot.

COMBINED

Pectoral tea: mix equal parts marshmallow, eucalyptus, and mullein. Place a teaspoon of this mixture in a cup, add boiling water, and let it steep for 10 minutes. Strain it and sweeten it. Drink 1 cup every 8 hours while it is hot, to relieve cold symptoms.

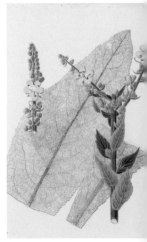

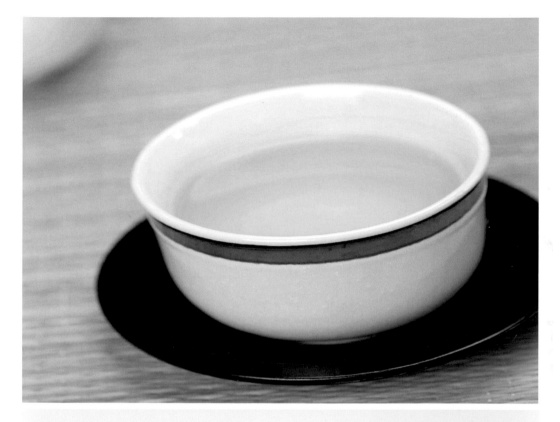

Precautions

It is not toxic, but its use is not recommended during pregnancy and lactation due to lack of research to ensure its safety.

Description

It is a herbaceous plant that grows to 5 feet (1.5 meters) high. Its leaves are large and plush with abundant woolly hairs. Its flowers are yellow and grow from thick spikes.

Cultivation

It grows in rocky terrain, dry grasslands, and arid parts of Europe. In Spain, it is more common in the north and in the east.

Harvesting

Mullein flowers and leaves are harvested from July to September, and they are left to dry in the sun or under artificial heat (95° to 104°F [35° to 40°C]); in a moist environment they turn brown and lose their effectiveness. They are kept in tightly closed jars, away from light and moisture.

Composition

It contains mucilage, flavonoids, iridoids, phenolic acids, saponins, simple sugars, and steroids.

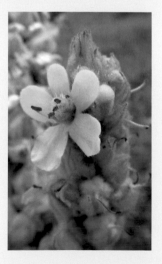

Greater plantain

(Plantago major)

Natural expectorant and laxative

Its name, "plantago" refers to the shape of its leaves which look as though they have been stepped on. It is in the same family as sand plantain. Since classical antiquity, it has been used for medicinal purposes. Currently, it is used as cough medicine and skin moisturizer.

When should you use it?

Thanks to its mucilage, greater plantain has an effective soothing, softening, and moisturizing effect on the respiratory mucosa to suppress cough. Therefore, it is a great cough medicine that clears out the chest and lungs. It is also anti-inflammatory and lipid lowering.

It is also useful when used in gargles made with the infusion to soothe your sore throat and to relieve canker sores. Also, thanks to its abundant mucilage,

it is a good remedy for chronic constipation and diarrhea. Furthermore, when used externally, its mucilage has a softening, emollient, and moisturizing effect on the skin. For this reason, it is very good for treating wounds, burns, and insect bites. Similarly, poultices made from its crushed leaves or cotton pads soaked in the infusion protect, moisturize, and soften dry or damaged skin.

Presentation

You can find its flower tops, dried and chopped, ready for making tea (1 teaspoon per cup), alone or combined with other plants in mixtures for treating colds and coughs. It is also possible to buy it in capsules (3 or 4 a day in 2 doses).

Remedies

BY ITSELF

Plantain infusion: mix a teaspoon of plantain in a cup of boiling water. Let it steep for 10 minutes and strain. Drink a cup every 8 hours, and you will get very good results for treating dry cough, bronchitis, and the common cold. It also has a mild laxative effect.

COMBINED

Expectorant tea: mix equal parts plantain, thyme, marshmallow, and eucalyptus. Place a teaspoon of this mixture in a cup and add boiling water. Let it steep for 10 minutes and strain. Drink 3 cups a day, while it is still hot. It is a cough medicine, expectorant, and antiseptic remedy that works well to relieve colds.

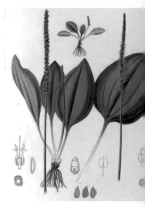

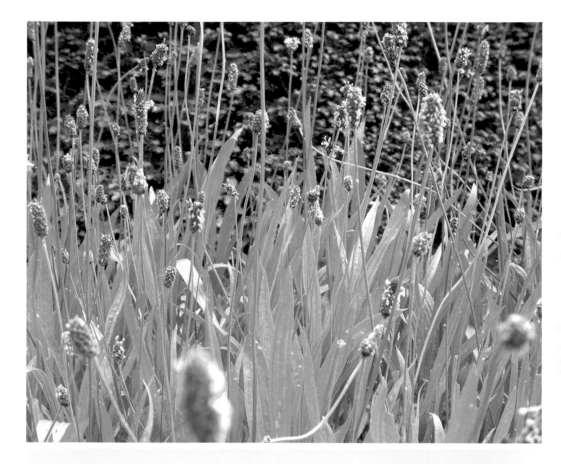

Precautions
It is a very safe choice, without toxicity, but it is not recommended during pregnancy and lactation and for small children.

Description
It is a perennial herbaceous plant with thick stems that can measure up to 2 feet (60 centimeters). A basal rosette made of large broad leaves grows from its stem. The leaves have parallel veins that converge at the tip. Its small white or purple flowers grow clustered together in a spike. Its fruit has several small seeds.

Cultivation
It grows wild in wet places, such as orchards and slopes.

Harvesting
Its flowering tops are harvested in late spring. It is left to dry in the shade, spread out in thin layers, and then kept in tightly closed containers, away from light and moisture.

Composition
It contains mucilage, pectins, tannins, flavonoids, phenolic acids, triterpenes, saponins, and mineral salts.

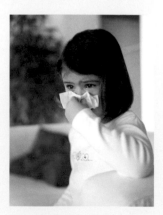

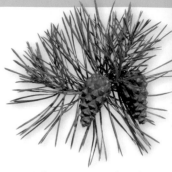

Scots pine

(Pinus sylvestris)

Ally against infections

Its buds give off an alluring scent due to its high essential oil content. This is precisely why it has soothing and antiseptic effects. It is a very effective remedy for those who often suffer from respiratory infections.

When should you use it?

Its expectorant and mucolytic properties are attributed to its richness in essential oil. It acts directly on the bronchial epithelium, exerting an irritant effect that increases the production of bronchial secretions, thereby making it easier to clear out the chest and lungs. It has an antiseptic effect on the respiratory system, which makes it an excellent remedy for winter respiratory infections; to relieve colds, bronchitis, and pharyngitis; and to soothe dry, irritating cough. Its antiseptic effect also acts on the kidney, so, although rarely, it is used to treat urinary disorders such as cystitis.

For external use, its essential oil has rubefacient properties that are effective in reducing inflammation and easing rheumatic pain.

Presentation

The most common way to use it is in vapor (2 tablespoons per quart (1 liter) of water) with dried and crushed bits of the plant. It is used to prepare infusions (1 teaspoon per cup). It can also be found in capsules and as an ingredient in herbal blends for infusion to treat respiratory conditions.

It is often used topically, especially its essential oil. An infusion made with its buds can be used for bathing. It is also an ingredient in ointments and gels for external use.

Remedies

BY ITSELF

Vapor: place 2 tablespoons of Scots pine in 1 quart (1 liter) of boiling water. Instead of using its buds, you can also prepare it with a few drops of essential oil. When it is ready, place your head over the container and inhale the vapor.

Bathing in Scots pine is good for relieving rheumatic pain because it has an anti-inflammatory and soothing effect. Prepare a decoction by placing a handful of buds in 2 quarts (liters) of water.

Boil it for half an hour and, once filtered, add it to hot bath water. Instead of using buds, use a few drops of its essential oil.

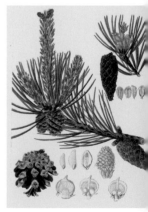

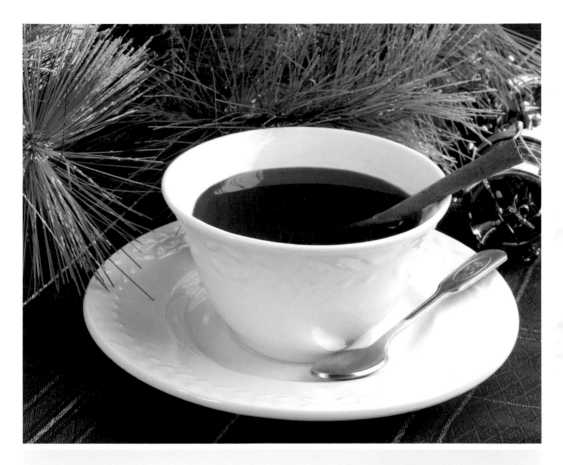

● Precautions
Using its essential oil is contraindicated during pregnancy and lactation, and for children under six. Use it with caution if you suffer from asthma because it can cause bronchoconstriction.

● Description
It is a tree with a straight and cylindrical trunk that grows to 33 to 98 feet (10 to 30 meters). Its needle-like, stiff, and blue-green leaves grow in intertwined pairs. It has yellow male inflorescences and female inflorescences that are its cones.

● Cultivation
It is of Eurasian origin. It grows in coastal areas and hills of northern Europe and also in the high mountain regions of the Mediterranean area.

● Harvesting
Its buds, bark, and resin are harvested by trained personnel.

● Composition
It contains essential oil, bitter substances, resin, and vitamins.

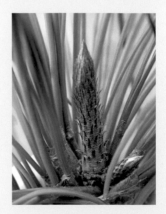

Lungwort

(Pulmonaria officinalis)

Relieves sore throat

This plant, rich in mucilage and allantoin is an excellent ally when a cold could not be prevented and you end up with hoarseness, cough, and sore throat. Lungwort provides relief, cleans your airways, and keeps them safe from infection.

When should you use it?

It is a gentle but effective expectorant whose mucolytic action soothes dry cough and sore throat. Its demulcent effect is also used to treat some gastrointestinal and urinary tract disorders. Applied externally, it moisturizes and softens the skin because of its emollient effect. Also, because it contains allantoin, it accelerates skin regeneration thereby shortening the healing time for wounds. By joining these two properties, this plant is very effective for curing inflamed skin lesions and burns.

Presentation

This plant is dried and cut for making infusions (2 teaspoons per cup) and decoctions. It is also mixed with other pectoral plants as treatments for colds, flu, and respiratory ailments.

Remedies

BY ITSELF
Pectoral infusion: place a teaspoon of the plant in a cup of cold water and boil it for a few minutes. Let it steep for 5 to 10 minutes and filter it. As an expectorant tea, sip it hot and sweetened with honey, several times a day.

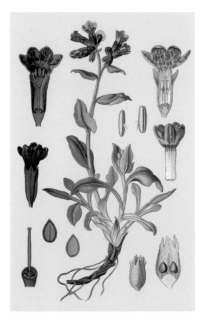

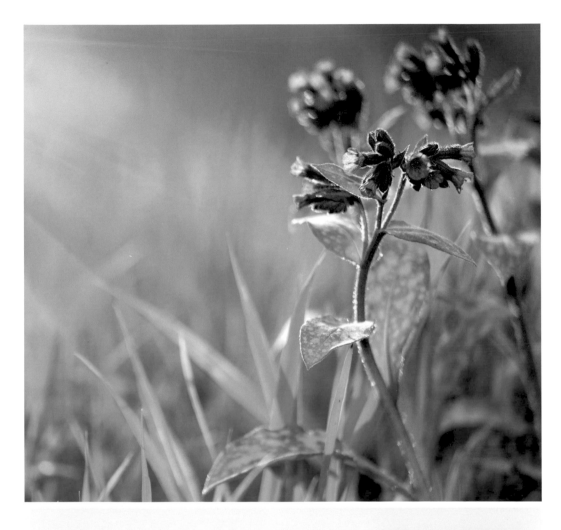

Precautions
Overall it is a remedy that has no toxicity, but its use is not recommended during pregnancy and lactation due to lack of research to ensure its safety.

Description
It is a plant that grows from to 6 in to 1 ft (15-30 cm) high. Its stems are erect, light green, and covered with glandular hairs. The basal rosette leaves have a long petiole, and its blue or purple flowers grow clustered together grouped in umbels.

Cultivation
Lungwort is native to Europe.

Harvesting
Its flowering tops are used.

Composition
It contains mucilage, phenolic acids, flavonoids, mineral salts, allantoin, and tannins.

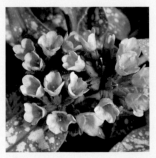

Elderberry

(Sambucus nigra)

Powerful remedy against colds

With its hollow branches, the Greeks created the sambuke, a musical instrument from which this plant derives its name. Its fruits have been used since ancient times as food; even now they are used to make delicious jams and juices. However, be careful not to confuse them with the fruits of dwarf elder, because although they are of the same family and share many properties, the fruits of the latter are highly toxic.

When should you use it?

It increases and thins bronchial secretions, facilitating their elimination. It causes profuse sweating (sudorific) and increased urination (diuretic), and exerts a strong purifying and decongestant action, so it is highly recommended for relieving colds and flu, and it is especially good for reducing fevers. It also works well to soothe dry cough. It also fights constipation because it has a laxative effect.

Its juice is popularly used as a remedy for sciatica and other joint pains. Its concentrated juice is used at high doses, as a purgative.

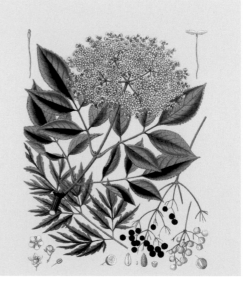

Presentation

Although it is rare in our country, the main way to use it is dried and ground for making infusions (1 or 2 teaspoons per cup), though you may find it in liquid extract (½ to ¾ teaspoon [1.5 to 3 milliliters] every 8 hours) and tinctures (½ to 1 teaspoon [2.5 to 7.5 milliliters] every 8 hours).

Remedies

BY ITSELF

Sudorific tea: place 2 teaspoons (10 grams) of elderberry in cold water and let it steep for several minutes. Then slowly bring it to boil and boil it briefly. Let it steep for 10 minutes and filter it. To treat fevers, drink a cup every 8 hours, and it is much more effective if you add lemon juice.

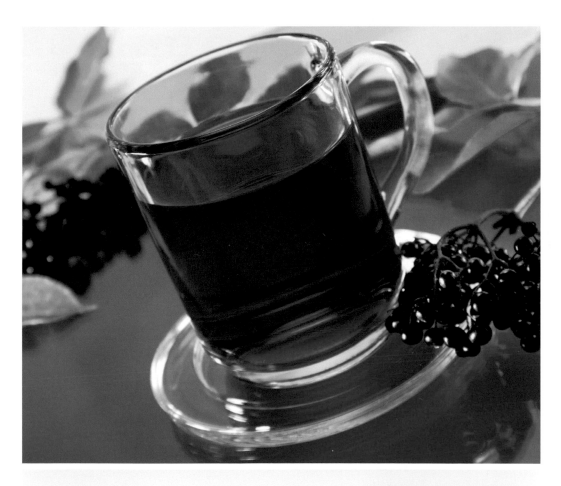

Precautions
It is a remedy devoid of toxicity, but its use is not recommended during pregnancy and lactation due to lack of research to ensure its safety.

Description
It is a large shrub, well branched, which can grow to 22 ft (7 m) high. Its leaves are deciduous, toothed, and dull green on top and bluish green on the underside. Its whitish flowers grow together in umbels. Its black or violet fruit has red juice.

Cultivation
It grows along roadsides, river-banks, and forests across Europe.

Harvesting
You can use its bark, leaves, roots, and inflorescences, but its fruits are the most commonly used. Its bark is harvested in spring, its leaves in the summer, and its flowers in late spring.

Composition
It contains flavonoids, essential oil, triterpenes, phenolic acids, mineral salts, mucilage, pectin, and tannins.

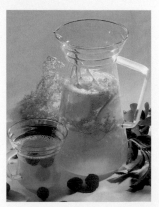

Absinthe wormwood

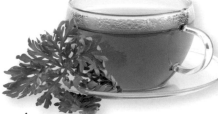

(Artemisia absinthium)

Stimulates the appetite

Known since ancient times, it was the Greeks who named it in honor of Artemis, goddess of fertility. This plant has been prized for its many healing applications, and its effect on appetite stimulation and digestion has contributed to its popularity as an ingredient for wines and liquors, most famously vermouth or absinthe. However, abuse of these drinks causes severe poisoning.

When should you use it?

Thanks to its bitter active ingredients, it helps stimulate appetite of those suffering from loss of appetite. It also has a tonic effect on the digestive system capable of improving poor digestion due to a deficiency of digestive juices and relieving its associated discomfort.

It is a good remedy because its anthelmintic action eliminates intestinal parasites, and its emmenagogue action helps regulate the menstrual cycle. In fact, it has been traditionally used by women who suffer irregular and painful periods.

Using this medicine does not cause the harmful effects of liqueurs made with it, among other things, because its strong bitter taste prevents us from taking too much.

Externally, absinthe is a good antiseptic and insecticide. Its infusion applied to the skin as a lotion repels mosquitoes, and placing dry absinthe in your closet, inside cloth pouches, keeps moths away from your clothing.

Presentation

Most commonly, you will find it dry and chopped for tea (1 teaspoon per cup of water), in liquid extract (¼ to ½ teaspoon [1 to 2 milliliters] every 8 hours), and tincture (10 to 30 drops every 8 hours).

Remedies

BY ITSELF

Digestive infusion: boil 3 tablespoons of the plant in 1 quart (1 liter) of water for 15 minutes. Let it steep for 5 minutes and strain. Drink 2 or 3 cups a day before meals if you want to stimulate your appetite, or after eating if you want to help your digestion.

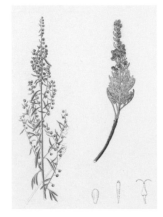

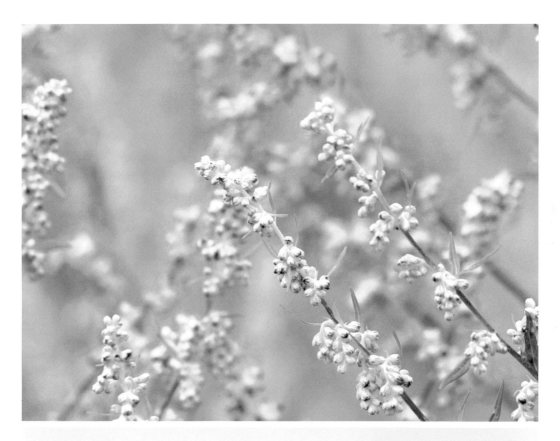

Precautions

It is not recommended for persons with epilepsy, for pregnant or nursing women, or for children under the age of 12.

Do not use for an extended period of time or at higher doses than recommended.

Description

It is a highly branched perennial plant that can grow up to 3 feet (1 meter) high. Its leaves are alternate, grayish green on top and silvery gray on the underside. Its small flowers are grouped in greenish yellow clusters.

Cultivation

It grows wild in Southern and Central Europe, North Africa, and Asia.

Harvesting

Its leaves and flowering tops are harvested before blooming. After the first year, they can be harvested twice, once in early summer and again in early winter.

Composition

It contains essential oil with a strong bitter flavor whose main component is thujone, but it also has lactones, flavonoids, tannins, phenolic acids, vitamins, and minerals.

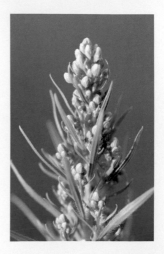

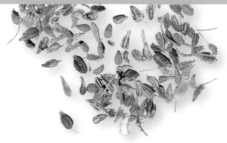

Anise

(Pimpinella anisum)

Condiment as an ally for digestion

Also known as "aniseed." Ancient Mediterranean civilizations used it both for its medicinal properties and to flavor foods and beverages. Today, its use has not changed much, and it is still used as a condiment in pastries, in some curries and seafood dishes, and in liqueurs, and it is a good remedy for digestion.

When should you use it?

It is a very effective remedy for reducing gas formation and facilitating its expulsion, due to its strong carminative effect. This, together with its gastrointestinal antispasmodic action, make it a very nice resource for relieving symptoms of difficult digestion, such as gases and painful bowel spasms, even in children. It also prevents bad breath.

But if that were not enough, it is a good expectorant and antiseptic recommended for treating dry cough, bronchitis, and pharyngitis. It also increases milk production in nursing mothers, and it regulates the menstrual cycle.

However, keep in mind that anise liqueur does not work like its infusions, quite the contrary. Drinking it excessively is not recommended because of its high alcohol content and because it may cause nerve damage.

Presentation

It is most traditionally sold dry, by weight or in tea-bags (1 teaspoon per cup). Its essential oil (0.1 milliliter per day, divided into 3 doses) is also very commonly used.

It is an ingredient in mixtures for infusion for improving digestion and it is also an ingredient in some special products (powdered) designed to relieve colic and other digestive disorders in infants and young children.

Remedies

BY ITSELF

Carminative infusion: place half a teaspoon in a cup and add boiling water. Let it steep for 10 minutes and strain. Drink a cup of this tea after meals to prevent gas and intestinal spasms attributed to poor digestion.

COMBINED

Digestive herbal tea: mix equal parts anise, fennel, and lemon balm. Place a teaspoon of this mixture in a cup and add boiling water. Let it steep for 10 minutes and strain it. Drink 3 cups after meals.

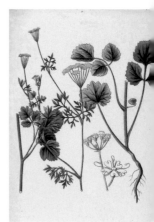

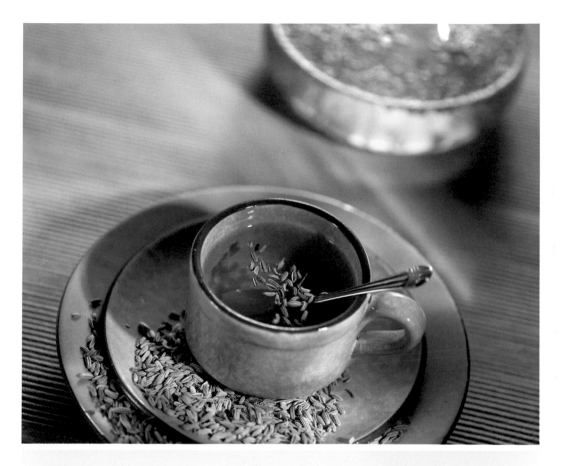

Precautions
It not recommended for use during pregnancy and lactation. Nor is it advisable to use its essential oil for children under 6 persons with epilepsy, for an extended period of time, or at higher doses than recommended.

Description
It is a herbaceous plant that grows to about 1.6 to 2.6 feet (50 to 80 centimeters) high. Its leaves are dark green and its whitish flowers grow clustered together. The fruit is an oval grain that exudes a very distinctive aroma.

Cultivation
It grows wild in Egypt, Greece, and the Middle East, but it is also cultivated in warm Mediterranean regions.

Harvesting
Its fruits are harvested from July to August, when they begin to turn light brown.

Composition
It contains essential oil, flavonoids, phenolic acids, coumarins, and triterpenes.

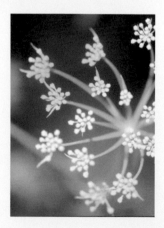

Fennel

(Foeniculum vulgare)

Goodbye gas

During the Middle Ages it was customary on the eve of the summer solstice to hang a fennel on the front door to ward off evil spirits, since it was considered a magical plant, capable of undoing witchcraft. Typically Mediterranean, its bulb is used as a vegetable, and its stems and leaves are used for flavoring. Its dried fruit is used as a condiment and for medicinal purposes.

When should you use it?

It has a remarkable ability to balance digestive functions. It stimulates digestion and has an effective carminative action, eliminating annoying intestinal gases that cause bloating and flatulence. It is also antispasmodic. It is especially suited for relieving spastic intestinal discomfort and colic in young children and babies. It also clears mucus from the respiratory tract with its expectorant and antiseptic properties, so it makes a good remedy for coughing and bronchitis.

Presentation

It is very commonly found in capsules and tablets, liquid extract (¼ to ¾ teaspoon [1 to 3 milliliters], before meals), in tinctures (1 teaspoon to 1 tablespoon [5 to 15 milliliters], before meals), syrups, and essential oil (0.1 to 0.6 milliliters every 24 hours).

It is also an ingredient in numerous mixtures for infusion, especially those preparations that are digestive, carminative, expectorant, and laxative. However, this plant is not recommended for infusion by itself, since its fruit is not effective without crushing, and once it is crushed, it loses its effectiveness very quickly.

Remedies

BY ITSELF

Digestive infusion: crush 1 to 3 teaspoons of its fruit and place them in a cup of boiling water. Let it infuse for about 10 minutes and then strain it. To alleviate gastrointestinal symptoms, drink a freshly prepared cup, 3 times a day, preferably after meals. For small children and infants, mix a small amount of infusion with milk.

COMBINED

Carminative tea: mix equal parts anise, lemon balm, and fennel. Place a teaspoon of this mixture in a cup of boiling water. Let it steep for 10 minutes and strain it. It relieves intestinal spasms, the feeling of fullness, and gets rid of gas.

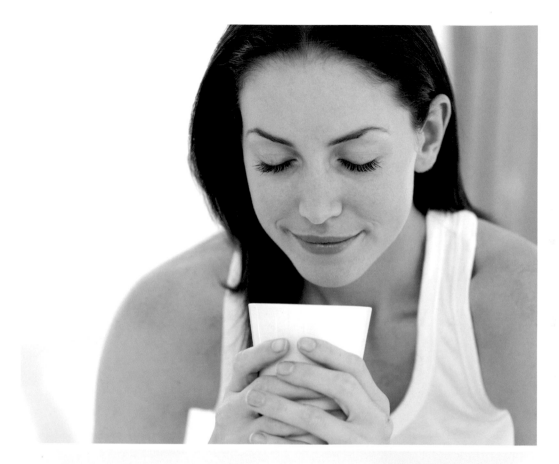

Precautions

It is not recommended to use during pregnancy and lactation. Its essential oil should not be given to young children, babies, or persons with epilepsy. Moreover, it is not advisable to use it for more than 2 weeks or in amounts higher than the recommended dose, due to possible toxicity.

Description

It is a herbaceous plant that can grow to more than 5 feet (1.5 meters) high. It is very aromatic, with feathery leaves and yellow flowers grouped in terminal umbels.

Cultivation

It usually grows in ditches, roadsides, fields, and uncultivated areas near the coast.

Harvesting

Its fruits are used for medicinal purposes, which are harvested starting in July. They can be slightly dried in the shade and then stored in tightly closed containers, away from light and moisture, for no longer than a year.

Composition

It contains essential oil, coumarins, and flavonoids.

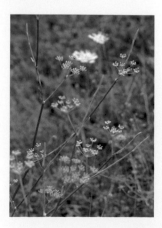

Chamomile

(Matricaria chamomilla)

Digestive balm

Even our grandparents used it, and today few plants are used more than chamomile. Its infusion, with soft and aromatic flavor, is the most consumed, and it is ideal at the end of especially heavy meals. This plant's virtues were known in ancient Egypt, where it was considered a sacred plant. This veneration remained among the Greeks and the Romans.

When should you use it?

Chamomile combines its power as a digestive stimulant with a natural sedative effect that makes it an excellent remedy to relieve nervous indigestion, abdominal pain, and gastrointestinal spasms. It is also good against colic, it helps stop diarrhea, relieves general feeling of malaise and nausea, and prevents vomiting. It is also recommended for hepatobiliary disorders, indigestion, and food poisoning. It is especially useful after a quick, heavy, and spicy meal because it decreases the feeling of abdominal heaviness and prevents the accumulation of gases and flatulence. Also, as a sedative plant, it calms the nerves and soothes the mind. For this reason, it is very effective for facilitating sleep in children and babies, as well as to mitigate menstrual cramps, morning sickness, tension headache, and irritability. Chamomile also has an emollient, soothing, and antiseptic action, so it is used externally to relieve skin irritations, eczema, and bites.

Presentation

Most commonly, you will find its dry flowers readily available for preparing an infusion (1 ½ teaspoons per cup of water), tincture (1 tablespoon [15 milliliters] every 8 hours), liquid extract (¾ teaspoon [3 milliliters] every 8 hours), and its essential oil, the latter preferably for external use.

Remedies

BY ITSELF

Digestive infusion: place a teaspoon and a half of flowers in a cup of water and boil for 2 minutes. Strain it and let it steep for 10 minutes. Drink it hot just after lunch to let your food settle, eliminate nausea, and prevent vomiting.

COMBINED

Carminative tea: mix equal parts chamomile, lemon balm, peppermint, valerian, and caraway. Mix a teaspoon of this herbal blend per cup of water and drink a cup after each meal.

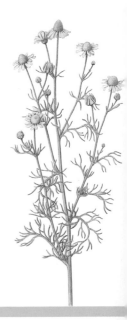

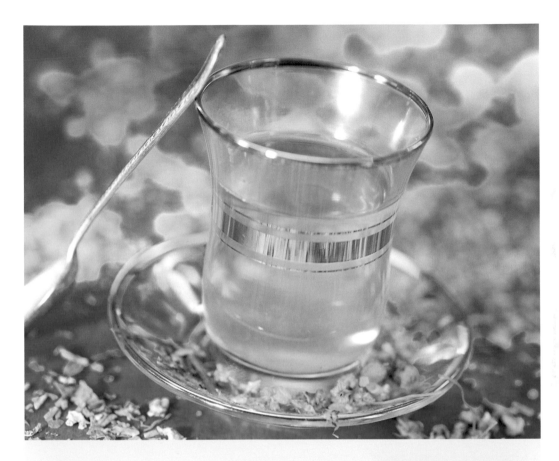

● Precautions

While chamomile is not toxic, its prolonged use or using too many flowers can cause gastrointestinal irritation and vomiting. Its essential oil should not be administered or topically applied to children under 6, persons with respiratory allergies, or those with known hypersensitivity to it.

● Description

Chamomile is a small herbaceous annual and branched plant. It has small flowers with white petals and yellow daisy-like buttons.

● Cultivation

In dry and sunny soil, roadsides, and fields throughout most of Europe. In Spain, it grows spontaneously and abundantly.

● Harvesting

Its flowering tops are harvested in spring. They are dried and kept in sealed containers. Chamomile normally grows wild, but it can easily grow at home without excessive care.

● Composition

Chamomile contains essential oil, flavonoids, mucilage, phenolic acids, and tannins.

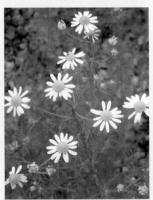

Peppermint

(Mentha piperita)

Refreshing and digestive tonic

There are many varieties, which even when hybridized they retain all their medicinal properties. Specifically, peppermint has been known since the 17th century, when it was developed through hybridization in England. It has a spicy taste and intense and fresh aroma, and it can be used both fresh and dried. It is a very versatile plant, highly valued for its use as a culinary condiment and for its medicinal use.

When should you use it?

This is a widely used remedy for proper digestion for the following reasons: it increases gastric juice secretion, so it helps in the digestive process; it makes it easier to digest fats because it increases bile production (it is cholagogue and choleretic); it has a strong carminative action and has a particularly intense intestinal antispasmodic effect. So, it is recommended as a treatment for gastritis and aerophagia, and especially to soothe intestinal cramping.

It has great results when mixed with other sedative plants. Peppermint essential oil can be inhaled (never for young children) and used as an expectorant and antiseptic nasal decongestant to treat some respiratory diseases. Applied externally, it is a very effective anti-rheumatic rubefacient. It is also useful for soothing itchy rashes and insect bites, because of its refreshing and antipruritic effect.

Presentation

Dry peppermint leaves are used for preparing infusions (1 teaspoon per cup) and decoctions. It is also available in liquid extract (½ teaspoon [2 milliliters] 2 to 3 times a day), tincture (2 teaspoons [10 milliliters] 2 to 3 times a day), and in essential oil (orally use 0.2 milliliter once a day, externally apply 5 to 15 drops several times a day). It is an ingredient in laxatives, anti-flatulent and digestive products, as well as in medication for regulating hepatobiliary functions. Its essence is used in pharmaceutical preparations.

Remedies

BY ITSELF

Infusion for digestive disorders: add a teaspoon of its leaves to a cup of boiling water. Let it steep for 10 minutes and strain. Drink 3 cups a day while it is freshly prepared and hot, and if possible, after meals.

COMBINED

Carminative tea: mix ½ cup (50 grams) hyssop, ½ cup (50 grams) orange blossom, and 1 cup (100 grams) peppermint. Add a teaspoon of this mixture to a cup of boiling water. Let it steep for 10 minutes and strain. Drink it after meals to prevent the formation of gases during digestion.

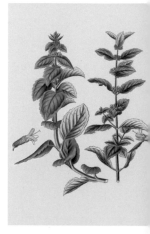

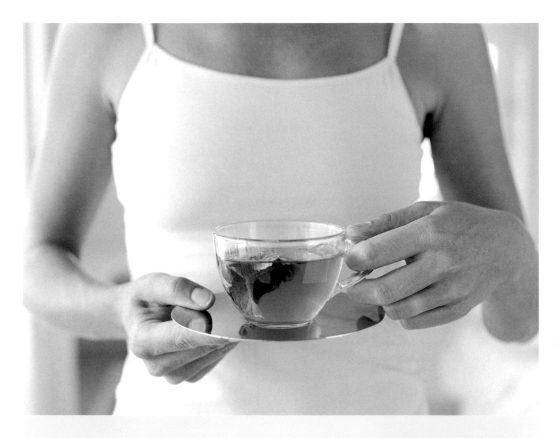

Precautions

It is contraindicated for persons suffering from biliary obstruction. If you suffer from gallstones, consult with a specialist before using it. Its essential oil in small children is to be used with caution, without exceeding the recommended dosage, and never apply it on the face.

Description

Peppermint is a herbaceous plant that grows up to 2.6 feet (80 centimeters). Its stalked leaves have toothed edges, and its flowers grow clustered together in elongated spikes. It gives off an intense and refreshing aroma.

Cultivation

Peppermint grows in all climates, but prefers moist soil. Although it can be in the sun, it grows better in the shade.

Harvesting

Its leaves are used both fresh and dry. They are harvested when the plant is about to bloom from late May to late July. At the start of autumn, they can be collected again. Dry them in the shade, in a well-ventilated area without heaping them too much. Then store them away from light and moisture in tightly closed containers.

Composition

It contains essential oil, flavonoids, phenolic acids, and triterpenes.

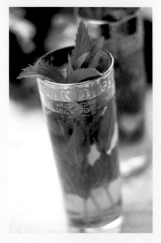

Papaya

(Carica papaya)

Digests protein and stimulates the defenses

Its fruit and the enzymes it contains have both been known and used for many years for their therapeutic properties. Aside from its medical use, papaya is highly regarded as food, for its use as a vegetable (unripe) or fruit (ripe), and in the food industry, where it is used to tenderize meat.

When should you use it?

Its proteolytic enzymes (such as papain) break down proteins quickly making the digestive process substantially easier. Therefore, it is used to improve heavy, slow digestion and eliminate gas, when there is a deficiency of gastric secretions or after overeating. Its vermifuge effect is useful for eliminating intestinal parasites. Also, recent studies demonstrate that its immunostimulatory activity is good for stimulating the body's natural defenses.

When externally applied, its anti-inflammatory action together with its proteolytic activity make it capable of lessening localized cellulite by splitting collagen fibers. It also works to heal wounds and skin lesions quickly.

In addition, papain is used in the technique known as chemonucleolysis, effective for treating herniated discs, which involves injecting papain in the nucleus of injured intervertebral discs.

Presentation

Besides as fruit, papaya can be consumed in capsules with dry extract. Papain is an ingredient in several pharmaceutical products.

Remedies

BY ITSELF

It is taken in capsules after meals, but you can also eat the fresh fruit because it is rich in beta carotene and vitamin C, and although its papain content is low, it tones digestion and is an excellent food for those suffering from digestive disorders.

In America, it is popularly used to eliminate intestinal parasites and diarrhea. Traditionally, its leaves have been used against malaria. The latex of its leaves is used to remove warts and for treating psoriasis.

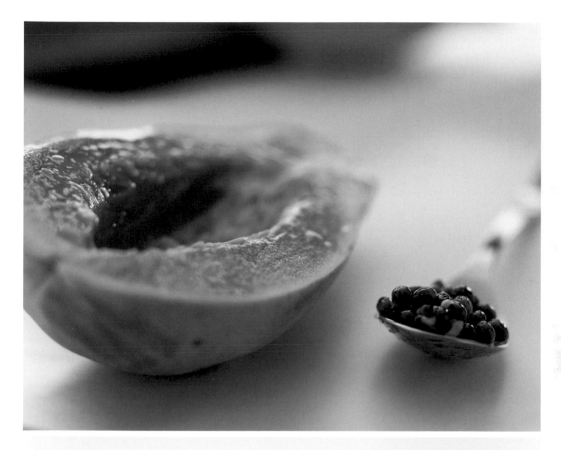

Precautions
Although it does not have any toxicity, be careful when using it during pregnancy and administering it to young children.

Description
It is a large shrub (9 to 32 feet [3 to 10 meters] tall), with a fleshy grayish trunk and a terminal cluster of leaves with long petioles. Its fruits are large ovoid berries that become yellow-orange once they ripen.

Cultivation
It appears to be native to Peru, although several authors believe that its origin is in Central America. Now it is cultivated in most tropical areas.

Harvesting
For medicinal purposes, its latex is obtained by making an incision on the fruit before ripening, and its leaves are also used.

Composition
It contains proteolytic enzymes such as papain, carbohydrates, proteins, organic acids, vitamins, and minerals.

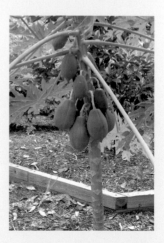

Shepherd's purse

(Capsella bursa-pastoris)

Stops bleeding and regulates the menstrual cycle

Its name comes from the fact that its fruit resembles a shepherd's bag. It has a long history of being used to stop bleeding, despite its unpleasant taste. In fact, even today it is still considered one of the best remedies for this purpose.

When should you use it?

It is hemostatic and vasoconstrictor, so taken orally it is a good remedy for regulating excessive menstrual bleeding and preventing epistaxis (nosebleeds). Applied externally as a compress, it is also antiseptic, so it is very suitable for treating minor skin wounds that bleed.

It is also recommended for people suffering from low blood pressure, especially thin women. It also has a useful diuretic effect for treating cystitis.

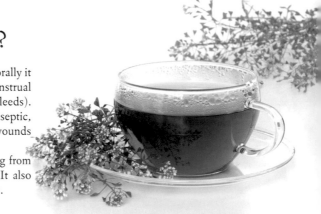

Presentation

You can find it in troches (dried and ground) for making infusions (1 ½ tablespoons [2 to 4 grams] per cup), although it is common to find it as an ingredient in mixtures for infusion, along with other related medicinal plants for treating menstrual disorders.

Remedies

BY ITSELF

Tea to control bleeding: add 2 or 3 teaspoons of the plant to a cup of boiling water. Let it steep for 10 to 15 minutes, then strain. It is best if you drink it after meals, up to 3 times a day. If bleeding persists, you should consult with a specialist.

COMBINED

Infusion for excessive periods: mix equal parts shepherd's purse, cypress, bitter orange, and butcher's broom. Add a tablespoon of this mixture to boiling water, let it steep for 10 minutes, then strain. You can sweeten it with sugar or honey. Drink 1 cup every 12 hours, preferably after meals.

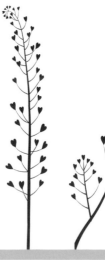

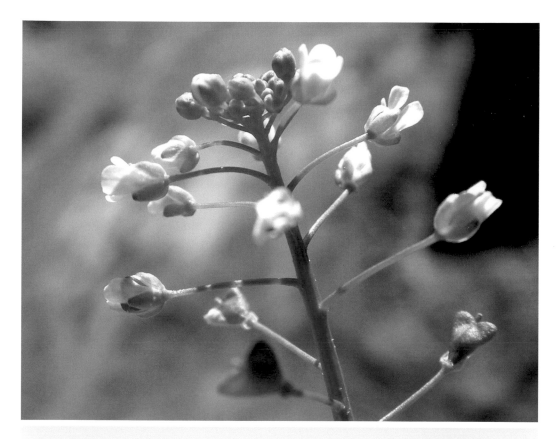

Precautions
It is not recommended for persons suffering from hypertension or for pregnant women.

Description
It is an annual plant that can grow up to 1.6 feet (50 centimeters). Its leaves form a rosette close to the ground. Its flowers are small and white. The most noticeable feature of this plant is its triangular and flat fruit that has a slightly salty taste. The fruit looks like a small purse carried by shepherds, hence its common name.

Cultivation
It is abundant in all kinds of environments altered by human activity, such as farm fields, edges of trails, and old walls (it is considered a "weed").

Harvesting
The parts of shepherd's purse that are used grow above ground. It can be found in bloom almost all year round, although it is more abundant in spring. After harvesting it fresh, it is dried in a ventilated place and then stored in tightly closed glass jars, away from dust and moisture.

Composition
It contains amine (tyramine, histamine, and choline), alkaloids, flavonoids, saponins, organic acids, and essential oil.

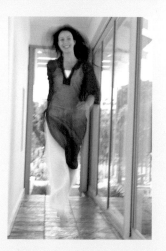

Horse-chestnut

(Aesculus hippocastanum)

Great ally of varicose veins

There is a very popular belief that exists among country people, whereby vein problems can be cured by simply carrying a few chestnuts inside your pocket. Today, it is well known that chestnut is an important alternative treatment for circulatory disorders.

When should you use it?

It increases the resistance of vein walls and reduces their permeability, so it invigorates blood circulation. It is also anti-inflammatory and prevents fluid retention. Therefore, it is a very useful treatment for varicose veins, tired legs, night cramps, and venous insufficiency. Its normal use is also an effective preventive measure for people who work long hours standing or have poor circulation problems.

Also, this plant relieves pain and reduces the size of hemorrhoids.

Moreover, horse-chestnut bark is rich in allantoin, which has emollient and anti-inflammatory properties, and it is very beneficial for skin care. If you add to this its venotonic power, it is not hard to understand why it is so often used as an ingredient for creams to treat wounds, sunscreens, and decongest skin creams. Horse-chestnut is also an ingredient in some shampoos because it stimulates capillary blood flow, which strengthens the scalp.

Presentation

It is easily available as capsules of powdered horse-chestnut, whose dosage is easy, practical, accurate, and indicated on the packaging. Also, you can buy different ointments and creams that contain extracts of this plant for varicose veins, tired legs, and hemorrhoids. Pharmacies carry medications that contain active ingredients extracted from this plant.

Remedies

BY ITSELF

The safest way to use it is by taking it orally in capsules or tablets, or applying it as topical cream. To improve hemorrhoids, take it orally, and make a decoction of its bark to prepare sitz baths with 2 cups (50 grams) of bark per quart (1 liter) of water. Boil it for 10 minutes and then strain.

COMBINED

It is an ingredient in many preparations, both orally and topically, along with other venous tonic plants such as witch-hazel, butcher's broom, ginkgo, and grape vine.

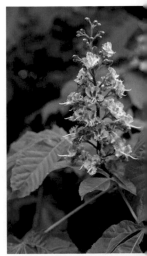

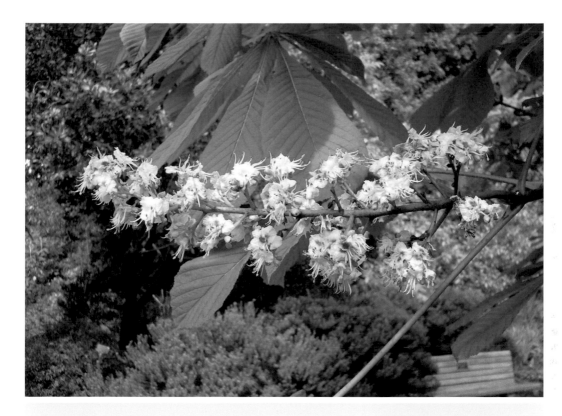

Precautions

At the recommended dose, it is not toxic, but it should not be used during pregnancy, breastfeeding, or if suffering from peptic ulcer or gastritis. Use horse-chestnut with caution if you are suffering from heart, liver, or kidney failure.

Description

It is a large deciduous tree with beautiful foliage. It grows to 98 feet (30 meters) high and lives for up to 300 years. Its leaves are palmate, large, with serrated edges, and grow in groups of 5 to 9. Its white flowers are grouped in clusters. Its large fruits are surrounded by thorns that are not too hard, and although they resemble chestnuts, they are not edible, and in fact, they could cause serious effects if ingested by children.

Cultivation

It is a very common tree in European and American parks and streets. It also grows in wild forests in mountainous regions.

Harvesting

The bark of young branches is harvested in spring and dried in the shade. Its seeds are collected from fruits that have fallen.

It contains saponins, flavonoids, tannins, coumarins, steroids, and allantoin.

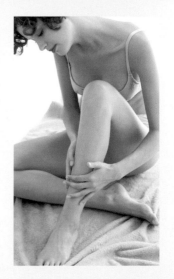

Ginkgo

(Ginkgo biloba)

Prevents circulatory disorders due to aging

This tree's longevity and resilience are a symbol of its beneficial properties for disorders that are common in old age. It has been used in Traditional Chinese Medicine since ancient times, and today, in addition to being the subject of numerous scientific research studies, it is a component of several pharmaceutical products.

When should you use it?

It acts on the entire circulatory system, improving both capillary circulation and venous circulation. Its vasodilatory and venotonic action protects the capillary veins, making it a very suitable remedy for cerebral circulatory insufficiency, varicose veins, phlebitis, tired legs, and swollen ankles.

It has been shown to contain antioxidant active ingredients that can prevent peroxidation of fats that circulate in the blood, thereby improving blood flow, especially microcirculation. Furthermore, it actives cerebral blood flow, so it can protect the brain from lack of blood supply. For example, it is beneficial for Alzheimer's disease and other dementias.

Although it has not been proven yet, using ginkgo may improve memory in healthy people and lessen PMS symptoms.

Presentation

Do not use ginkgo leaves in teas and other homemade preparations, because they do not provide the necessary concentration for it to be effective. It is better to use it in capsules, tablets, liquid extract, and tincture. Although the dosage is already indicated for such products, it is best to consult with a physician. In pharmacies you can find prescribed medication with ginkgo as an ingredient.

Remedies

BY ITSELF

Orally, it is preferable to use it in premeasured doses. For external use to improve circulation in the hands and feet, you can prepare hand baths and foot baths with an infusion of up to 3 cups (100 grams) of ginkgo leaves per quart (1 liter) of water. Apply it warm or hot once or twice a day.

COMBINED

Ginkgo is very often combined with grape vine, butcher's broom, fennel, hawthorn, oats, Saint John's wort, Siberian ginseng, and garlic.

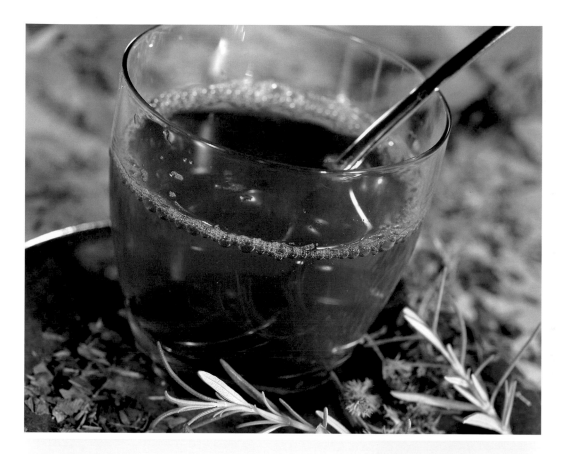

Precautions
Ginkgo is contraindicated for hypertension, diabetes, children under the age of 12, and during pregnancy and lactation. Keep in mind that it interacts with oral anticoagulants.

Description
It is an archaic tree that grows up to 98 feet (30 meters) high. It is dioecious (distinct male and female organisms), with deciduous thick and elastic leaves that are divided into two lobes. Its fruits are yellow drupes that are edible when they are fresh, but they are smelly once they ripen.

Cultivation
It is native to China, Japan, and Korea, but it has now spread as an ornamental tree for parks and public roads in temperate regions of Europe and America.

Harvesting
Its leaves are collected in autumn, and its active ingredients are extracted for medicinal purposes. Its dry leaves are then chopped and stored in air-tight containers.

Composition
Among other things, it contains flavonoids, lactones, phenolic acids, tannins, organic acids, and steroids.

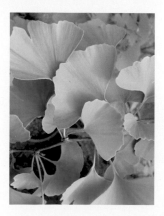

Witch-hazel

(Hamamelis virginiana)

Tones the veins and pampers your skin

The fruits of this tree, like hazelnuts, are unique in that they burst noisily when they ripen, which may be the reason Indians who used its leaves believed that this tree was haunted.

When should you use it?

This plant has the capacity to contract vein walls and reduce their permeability, so that it invigorates blood circulation (venotonic) making it a useful remedy for varicose veins, phlebitis, tired legs, and hemorrhoids. It is also anti-inflammatory and anti-diarrheal. Applied externally, it has healing, antiseptic, and astringent actions, so it is very effective for protecting and decongesting the skin and for healing small injuries and minor burns. It has ocular decongestant effect and can be used as eye drops to wash and relax your eyes, for combating conjunctivitis caused by environmental pollution and alleviating eye fatigue caused by excessive visual effort.

Presentation

You can buy it dried and chopped for making tea (1 teaspoon per cup) or decoctions, in capsules (the manufacturer indicates the dose), as liquid extract (½ to ¾ teaspoon [2 to 4 milliliters] every 8 hours), and tincture (½ to ¾ teaspoon [2 to 4 milliliters] every 8 hours). It is also the main ingredient in some suppositories, creams, and gels to tone the veins and for skin-care treatment, for which the manufacturer indicates its administration, dosage, and expiration date. Pharmacies carry eye drops with witch-hazel for tired and irritated eyes.

Remedies

BY ITSELF

Venotonic infusion: add a teaspoon of witch-hazel to a cup of boiling water. Let it steep for 10 minutes and strain. If you prefer, sweeten it with sugar or honey. Drink up to 3 cups a day, preferably after meals. This infusion will strengthen vein walls, improving circulation.

COMBINED

As oral treatment for hemorrhoids, it is usually mixed with other plants like plantain, ginkgo, and grape vine. For external use, it is mixed with butcher's broom and marigold.

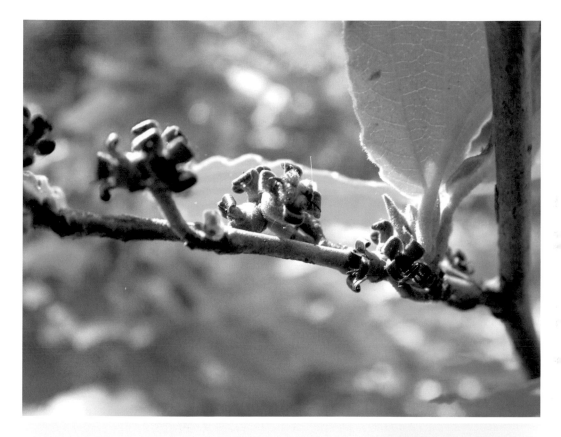

Precautions
It is contraindicated for peptic ulcer, gastritis, and during pregnancy and lactation. If you are using it as a treatment for diarrhea and it continues for 3 or 4 days, consult with a physician before continuing to use this remedy.

Description
This is a shrub that grows to 16 feet (5 meters) high. Its leaves are alternate, oval, and its very fragrant flowers have four yellow, tongue-shaped petals.

Cultivation
It is native to the west coast of the United States and Canada. It is currently grown as an ornamental tree in Europe.

Harvesting
Witch-hazel leaves and bark are normally used dry. Its leaves are harvested during the summer, then dried in the shade as quickly as possible, and kept in sealed jars away from light and moisture.

Composition
Its chemical constituents include tannins, flavonoids, and essential oil.

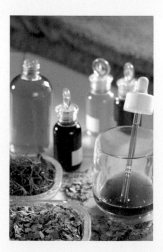

Sweet clover

(Melilotus officinalis)

Prevents thrombosis

This deliciously aromatic plant has been used for medicinal purposes since ancient times. Beneficial virtues to relieve the eyes were attributed to it, so until not long ago it was common to use it for eye baths and compresses. Even now, popular medicine credits it with having diuretic and antispasmodic properties. Currently, it has been shown to have valuable venotonic activity.

When should you use it?

It invigorates blood circulation and activates the lymphatic system. On the one hand, it increases venous flow, improving microcirculation while decreasing capillary permeability, and on the other, it increases lymph flow and accelerates the absorption of edema (fluid retention). It is an effective remedy for alleviating conditions associated with chronic venous insufficiency, such as pain and heaviness in the legs, night cramps in the calves, itching, and swelling. It is also used to treat hemorrhoid pain, itching, and inflammation. It also has a slight anticoagulant effect, thereby decreasing blood viscosity, preventing thrombosis.

Used externally, it has anti-inflammatory action, and it accelerates healing and tissue regeneration. It is effective for relieving bruises and sprains.

Presentation

It is not very common in our country, but you can find the dry and crushed plant ready for preparing infusions (2 teaspoons per cup of water), which is the most traditional way of using it. It is also possible to find it in capsules and as liquid extract (20 to 40 drops, 2 or 3 times a day). It is also an ingredient in oral and topical medicines for venous insufficiency.

Remedies

BY ITSELF

Vasoprotective infusion: place 1 or 2 teaspoons of sweet clover in a cup of boiling water. Let it steep for 15 minutes and strain. To relieve pain and itching in the legs, drink 2 to 3 cups a day, preferably after meals. This same infusion can be applied externally in the form of baths and compresses.

COMBINED

To activate blood circulation, sweet clover works well when combined with blueberry, witch-hazel, grape vine, ginkgo, and bitter orange, both in teas and in capsules.

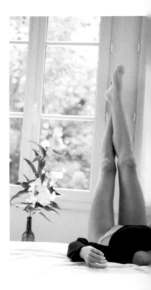

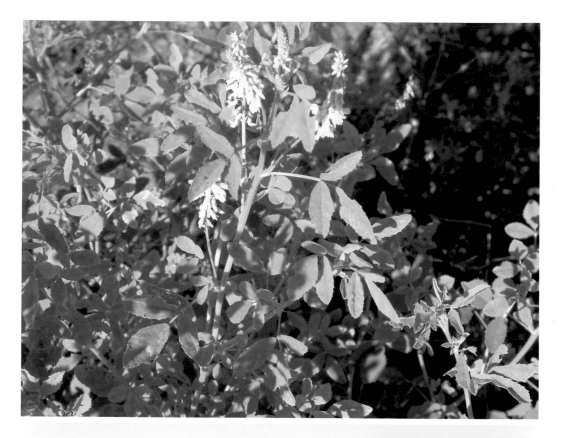

Precautions

It is not recommended during pregnancy or lactation, or for children under the age of 12. For persons suffering from liver failure, consult with a specialist before using. It is not recommended for treatments lasting longer than 3 months.

Description

It is an herbaceous plant with trifoliate leaves and small yellow flowers in elongated clusters. Its fruit is a small ovoid pod.

Cultivation

It is found in most of Europe, except in the far south. It grows on roadsides, in meadows, and generally in argillaceous and saline soil.

Harvesting

Its flowering tops are harvested when its flowers are fully developed, starting in May. They have to be dried as quickly as possible, in the shade, and, once dried, they are chopped and stored in tightly sealed jars away from light.

Composition

It contains saponins, flavonoids, coumarins, and their derivatives.

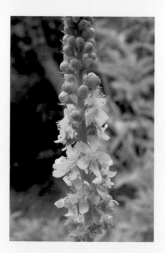

Butcher's broom

(Ruscus aculeatus)

Tonic for veins

Butcher's broom is well known because it is often used as a symbol of prosperity at Christmastime. In some places, its young shoots are eaten; they are similar to asparagus, but their taste is much more bitter. However, its red berries are never eaten because they are toxic.

Since long ago, it has been used as a diuretic, even though it has not been demonstrated to have such effect. However, it has been demonstrated that it tones and stimulates venous circulation.

When should you use it?

It protects and strengthens vein walls thereby increasing their resistance and reducing their permeability while strengthening venous circulation. It is also anti-inflammatory, diuretic, and prevents water retention. Thanks to all these properties, butcher's broom is a great remedy for relieving venous disorders affecting the legs, such as varicose veins, or illnesses caused by using the contraceptive pill. It is also a good treatment option for hemorrhoids and to relieve tired legs.

It can also be used to decongest and lessen redness and blotchiness of the hands.

Presentation

You can find the root, dried and chopped, ready for making tea (1 teaspoon per cup) and decoctions, in capsules (its dose is indicated by the manufacturer), liquid extract (30 drops 3 times a day), and tinctures (1 to 2 teaspoons [5 to 10 milliliters] 3 times a day). It is an ingredient in creams and suppositories to relieve poor circulation in the legs and to treat hemorrhoids.

Remedies

BY ITSELF

It works best when it is simultaneously used internally and externally. Orally, it can be taken as a tea or in capsules, and it can be applied externally in the form of suppositories and creams. For external use, you can prepare a decoction by slicing a piece of butcher's broom root and boiling it in with some water for 10 minutes, then let it sit and filter it so you can use it as a compress.

COMBINED

Venotonic infusion: mix equal parts butcher's broom root, ginkgo, witch-hazel, and yarrow. Place a teaspoon of this mixture in a cup and add boiling water. Let it steep for 10 minutes and strain. Drink it after meals. It improves problems associated with poor venous circulation in the legs.

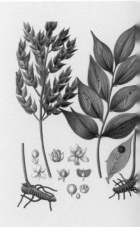

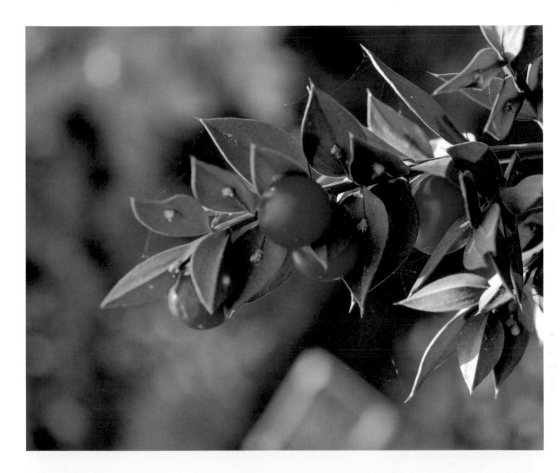

Precautions
Although it is a fairly safe remedy, it is not recommended for use during pregnancy or lactation, or for children under the age of 12.

Description
Butcher's broom is a perennial shrub. At first glance, its small leaves seem very sharp, but they are actually modified leaf-shaped stems with hard and sharp edges.

Cultivation
It grows abundantly in much of Europe, in forests, hedges, and even roadsides. It is a nice plant to have in the garden, if you do not care about its thorny edges.

Harvesting
The rhizome and root are the parts of the plant that are used. They are harvested in autumn and dried in the shade. They are stored in tightly closed containers away from light and moisture until they are used.

Composition
It contains tannins, flavonoids, saponins, and essential oil.

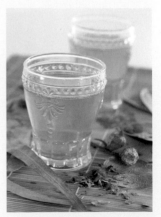

Grape vine

(Vitis vinifera)

Increases elasticity of the veins and protects them

It is one of the plants with the greatest tradition in the history of agriculture. Wine is extracted from it, it gives us delicious and healthy grapes to eat, and its leaves are used in herbal medicine as a remedy for venous insufficiency.

When should you use it?

It is a powerful venotonic, vasoprotector, and antioxidant remedy. First, it strengthens vein walls so that they swell less, and secondly, it prevents the degradation of elastin and collagen, giving greater elasticity to the vessels. It also reduces the permeability of blood capillaries thereby reducing edema (fluid retention). If to all this you add its vasodilating action, which facilitates blood flow, it is easy to see that this is an excellent remedy to improve poor circulation in the lower extremities and thus prevent the onset of varicose veins, phlebitis, and capillary fragility, or improve their symptoms. It also relieves leg pain and itching, and muscle cramps caused by poor circulation. It is even an effective remedy to treat chilblains.

Also, with these same properties, it soothes and relieves painful hemorrhoids.

Externally, anti-inflammatory and antioxidant properties are used for skin care.

Presentation

It is easy to find its leaves, dried and chopped (troches) ready for preparing tea (1 teaspoon per cup). You can also buy grape vine liquid extract (1 teaspoon [5 milliliters] per day divided into 3 doses), capsules with dry leaves or powder (dosage indicated by the manufacturer), and tincture. Additionally, grape vine is an ingredient of many preparations, for both oral and external use, where it is mixed with other venotonic plants.

Remedies

BY ITSELF

Decoction to relieve chilblains: mix a teaspoon of leaves per cup of water, boil it for 10 minutes, and let it steep for another 10 minutes. Strain it and once it is warm, use it to wash your feet or hands. Use it for 5 minutes, 3 times a day. Dip your legs in this decoction to relieve leg pain.

COMBINED

Invigorating infusion for varicose veins: mix equal parts witch-hazel, butcher's broom, goldenrod, and grape vine. Add 1 teaspoon of this mixture to a cup of boiling water and let it steep for 10 minutes. Then strain it and sweeten it with honey or sugar, if you prefer. To improve circulation, drink 3 cups a day after meals.

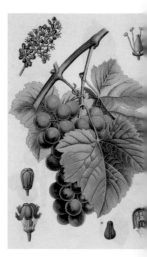

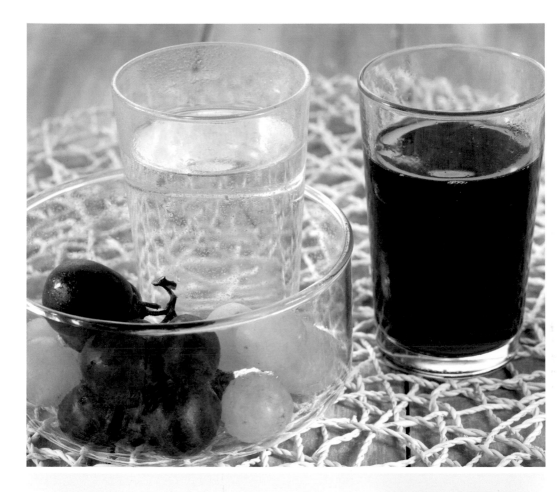

Precautions
It is a very safe choice, without toxicity. However, it is not recommended that treatment exceed a period of 3 months.

Description
It is a climbing shrub with small flowers that are grouped in clusters. Its fruits are black, yellow, or green grapes.

Cultivation
This plant is native to Asia Minor, but it has spread throughout all Mediterranean countries, where it is grown extensively.

Harvesting
For phytotherapeutic purposes, its leaves are harvested in the fall. Once dried, they are stored in tightly closed containers away from light and moisture.

Composition
It contains flavonoids, tannins, organic acids, phenolic acids, and, in particular, resveratrol.

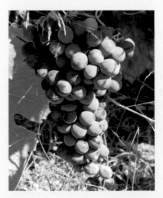

Chicory

(Cichorium intybus)

Stimulates appetite and improves digestion

This plant has popularized vegetables such as escarole or endive. Its leaves are used for both culinary and medicinal purposes. Furthermore, its dried root can be a healthy coffee substitute. As a vegetable, it is very easy to prepare it. Pair with other foods that counteract its particular bitter taste to make delicious and refreshing salads with nutritional and medicinal properties.

When should you use it?

Whether fresh or dry, use it before meals—its components help to stimulate the appetite of children and adults, and strengthen the digestive system. Thanks to its lactucopicrin, responsible for the bitter taste of chicory leaves, it also has a cholagogue effect; that is, it facilitates emptying the gall bladder and therefore improves food digestion. Thus, it clears the liver and improves its functions. Chicory is recommended for those suffering from gallbladder and liver disorders and slow digestion.

Its mild laxative action also treats chronic constipation, and its mild diuretic effect helps prevent water retention. Dried chicory root is used as a coffee substitute, with the advantage that it is a digestive infusion without any stimulants.

Presentation

Use its freshly picked leaves in salads or fresh juice. Its juice is very bitter but very effective for stimulating appetite. Use its fresh or dried root for preparing decoctions (2 teaspoons per cup). The root is also available dried and crushed for preparing coffee substitute (dried, roasted, and ground). It can also be found in liquid extract (2 to 6 drops per day split into multiple doses).

Remedies

BY ITSELF

Digestive decoction: mix a cup of water with 2 teaspoons of chicory root and boil it for 5 minutes. Let it steep for 10 minutes and strain. Drink up to 3 cups a day, before meals, to stimulate your appetite and digest your food well.

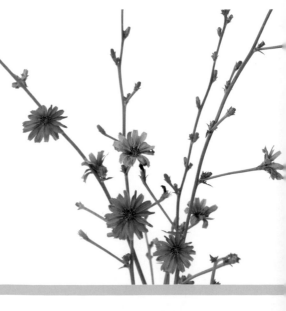

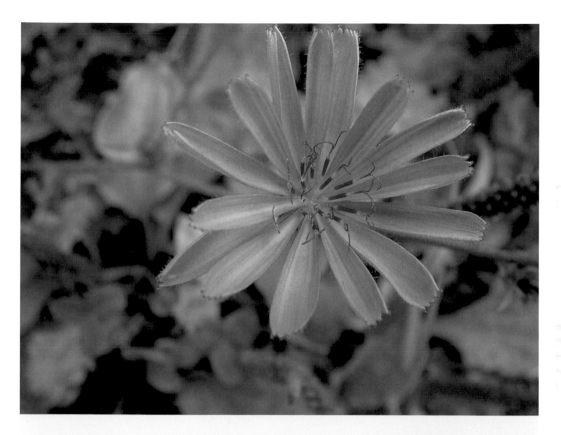

● Precautions
If you are suffering from gallstones, consult with your doctor before using it.

● Description
Chicory is an herbaceous plant with upright stems and beautiful light blue flowers whose petals end in five fine points. They are closed at night or in bad weather. All parts of the plant, including the latex, taste bitter.

● Cultivation
It grows isolated and in groups and is very common in roadsides, walls, embankments, and dry soils in temperate zones of Europe and America.

● Harvesting
Its leaves are harvested before the plant blooms from June to September, and the roots are collected in October. The root is dried and cut into ¼- to ⅓-inch (1- to 2-centimeter) pieces. Once dried, it is stored in opaque, tightly closed containers away from light. Since its leaves are usually eaten fresh, keep them in the warmest part of the refrigerator in a perforated plastic bag so that they can continue to "breathe."

● Composition
It contains inulin, intybin, and lactucopicrin as well as tannins, mineral salts, and vitamins.

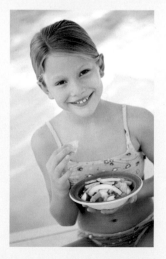

Artichoke

(Cynara scolymus)

Cares for the liver and lowers cholesterol

Although previously it had not been given much importance as a medicinal plant, from the twentieth century on, it has begun to enjoy a reputation as a remedy for liver and biliary disorders. In fact, some of its active ingredients are included in pharmaceutical products for liver health.

When should you use it?

Both its leaves and stem, whether fresh or dried, are an excellent remedy for liver damage and biliary diseases, besides being hepatoprotectve (that is, it protects the liver from toxins). It is cholagogue and choleretic, which promotes good digestive functions.

It is a highly recommended remedy for slow digestion and liver failure. It is also diuretic, purifying, and contributes to the elimination of urea, so it is beneficial for those suffering from kidney failure. Artichoke also helps lower blood cholesterol levels.

Presentation

The most common way of benefitting from its medicinal properties is by eating fresh artichoke heads. Besides eating artichokes, you can prepare fresh juice using fresh leaves; drink it immediately, because you can only keep it for a few hours.

For making infusion (1 teaspoon per cup) you can easily find its leaves, dried and chopped. Use it in tincture (1 teaspoon [6 milliliters] every 8 hours), ampoules (with the liquid extract), and capsules (dry artichoke or extract powder).

Remedies

BY ITSELF

Infusion for proper digestion: add a teaspoon of leaves to a cup of boiling water. Let it steep for 10 minutes and strain. Drink it half an hour before meals. It can be sweetened with sugar or honey.

COMBINED

Regulatory hepatic infusion: mix equal parts boldo, artichoke, and thistle. Mix a teaspoon of this mixture per cup of boiling water and let it steep for 10 minutes. Then strain it and drink 3 cups a day, half an hour before meals.

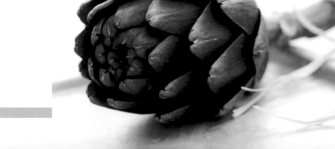

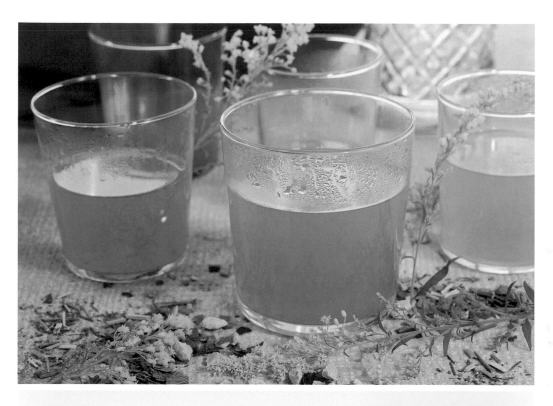

● **Precautions**
Although it is a remedy without toxicity, is not recommended for gallstones without the supervision of a specialist. Nor is it recommended for infants. It is contraindicated for persons suffering from bile duct obstruction.

● **Description**
It grows up to 5 feet (1.5 meters) high. Its grayish green leaves are large and very segmented. Its violet-blue flower heads are surrounded by bracts (false leaves), on which the edible part rests.

● **Cultivation**
Although it is typical of the Mediterranean countries, where it is grown in gardens, nowadays it is grown in temperate regions around the world.

● **Harvesting**
Its leaves, preferably those grown in the first year, stem, and flower heads (artichokes) are harvested from autumn to spring (it is harvested in multiple steps). Its leaves are dried in the sun and stored in glass jars in a dark and dry place for no longer than 1 year.

● **Composition**
It contains cynarin, flavonoids, essential oil, triterpenoids, tannins, steroids, and polysaccharides (inulin and mucilage).

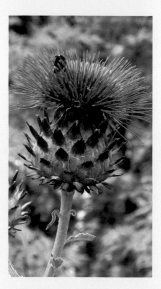

Boldo

(Peumus boldus)

Great friend of the gallbladder

The native people of Chile, in the Andes, used boldo leaves as a remedy for stomach and digestive disorders. Today, it is a very common remedy in pharmacies and health food stores. In fact, it is one of the most widely used medicinal plants for pharmaceuticals that treat gallbladder disorders.

When should you use it?

This remedy's most important virtues are its ability to protect the liver and its effectiveness in increasing the production of bile in the liver (choleretic effect) and to facilitate emptying of the gallbladder (cholagogue effect). Boldo leaves are especially recommended for problems with gallbladder function, such as slow or difficult digestion, bloating, and bad taste in the mouth (bitterness), caused by malfunctioning gallbladder. In addition, it is a gentle yet effective laxative that helps fight chronic constipation.

Presentation

Most commonly, dried and chopped boldo leaves are used for preparing infusions (one teaspoon per cup). But it is very often combined with other choleretic and cholagogue plants or laxatives. It is also sold in capsules in dosages recommended by the manufacturer.

Furthermore, its active ingredients are extracted from boldo bark and used in certain pharmaceuticals for treating liver and gallbladder diseases.

Remedies

BY ITSELF

Infusion for biliary dyspepsia: place a teaspoon of leaves in a cup of boiling water. Let it steep for 10 minutes and strain. Drink up to 3 cups a day, half an hour before meals.

COMBINED

Liver decongestant tea: mix equal parts boldo, fumitory, rosemary, dandelion, and anise. Place 2 teaspoons of this mixture in a cup of boiling water. Let it steep for 10 minutes and strain. To improve liver function, drink up to 3 cups before meals.

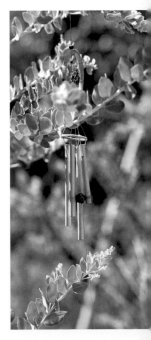

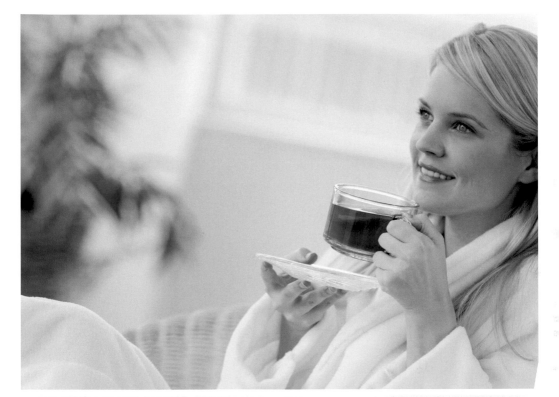

Precautions

It should not be used during pregnancy or lactation, for young children, or for persons suffering from bile duct obstruction or severe liver disease. Although boldo preparations are good for liver function, do not ingest it in excess. Do not use boldo as a treatment for longer than 4 weeks, and do not exceed the recommended doses.

Description

Boldo is a tree or shrub that grows up to 16 feet (5 meters) tall, with rough elliptical leaves. Its flowers are white or yellowish. The whole plant gives off a pleasant scent similar to peppermint.

Cultivation

It grows wild in dry and sunny slopes of Chile and the Andean regions of South America, but it is also grown in Italy and North Africa.

Harvesting

Its leaves are harvested from December to March. Active ingredients are also extracted from its bark. The leaves become brittle when dried, so handle them gently.

Composition

Its main active components include alkaloids, essential oil, flavonoids, coumarins, and tannins.

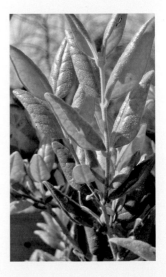

Milk thistle

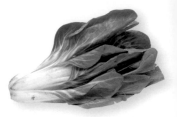

(Silybum marianum)

Potent liver regenerator

Thistle is native to Mediterranean temperate zones, where it has been used since ancient times. In many regions, it is a traditional winter vegetable served at Christmas parties. It has a delicate, sweet, and slightly bitter flavor. Although it is not very rich in nutrients, it provides other active components, such as silymarin and inulin, to which it owes its medicinal properties.

When should you use it?

It is one of the most effective remedies for protecting and healing the liver because it contains silymarin, a substance capable of regenerating liver cells damaged by toxins and relieving liver tissue inflammation. Boldo is therefore an excellent remedy for hepatitis and liver failure. It is also used to treat liver disorders caused by insufficient bile secretion, such as gallstones and biliary dyspepsia. It has good hepatoprotective effects to relieve symptoms related to overeating, and alcohol and drug abuse. As if this were not enough, thistle also stimulates appetite, it is diuretic, has a mild laxative effect, and helps reduce high cholesterol levels because it has lipid-lowering activity. In addition, it can be used externally as an anti-inflammatory to relieve sunburn and dermatitis.

Presentation

It is available in tinctures (¼ to ½ teaspoon [1 to 2 milliliters] every 8 hours), liquid extract (20 to 30 drops, 2 or 3 times a day), and dried and ground for preparing infusions. It is pulverized into capsules whose dosage is indicated by the manufacturer. Moreover, silymarin is extracted from the fruits of milk thistle, and it is an ingredient in multiple liver medications.

Remedies

BY ITSELF

Decoction to maintain a healthy liver: add a teaspoon and a half of thistle to a cup of water and boil it for 2 minutes. Let it steep for 5 minutes and strain. Drink 2 or 3 cups a day before meals for good liver function.

COMBINED

Hepatoprotective tea: Mix equal parts milk thistle, rosemary, and boldo. Add a teaspoon of this mixture to a cup of boiling water, and let it steep for 10 minutes. Strain it and drink it before meals. This tea helps to relieve the liver after overeating.

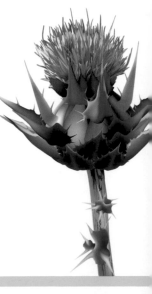

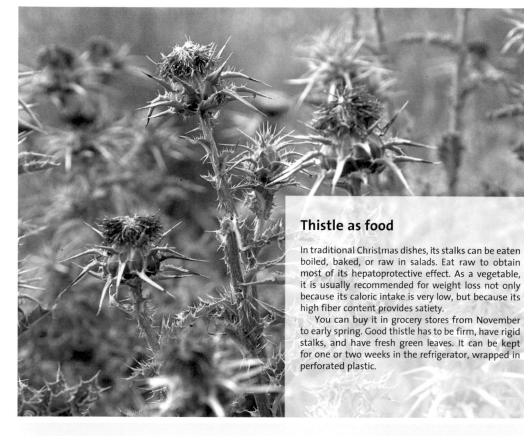

Thistle as food

In traditional Christmas dishes, its stalks can be eaten boiled, baked, or raw in salads. Eat raw to obtain most of its hepatoprotective effect. As a vegetable, it is usually recommended for weight loss not only because its caloric intake is very low, but because its high fiber content provides satiety.

You can buy it in grocery stores from November to early spring. Good thistle has to be firm, have rigid stalks, and have fresh green leaves. It can be kept for one or two weeks in the refrigerator, wrapped in perforated plastic.

Precautions

Milk thistle should not be used during pregnancy or lactation, or for persons suffering from bile duct obstruction. It is also contra-indicated for persons allergic to milk thistle or other species of the Compositae family.

If you have gallstones, use milk thistle with great caution, and consult with a specialist.

Description

It is a vigorous plant that can grow up to 6.5 feet (2 meters) high. Its large and thorny leaves are peculiarly marbled with white. Its pink or purple flower heads are large. Its fruits are hard and dark.

Cultivation

It is a Mediterranean species that grows wild in dry, sunny, and rocky terrain.

Harvesting

For medicinal purposes, its fruits are harvested in early spring.

Composition

Its active ingredients include flavanolignanes (silymarin), mucilage, flavonoids, saponins, and phytosterols.

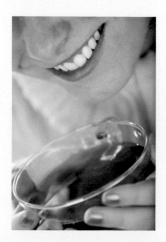

Dandelion

(Taraxacum officinale)

Great ally of the liver and kidneys

It is a very common plant that has many beneficial health properties, but it is most known as an ordinary "weed." Its fresh leaves can be eaten in salads, and their great purifying power makes dandelion an essential element in detoxifying cleanses. It is a great ally for liver and kidney health, but it is also essential in weight loss because of its low caloric content and satiating effect.

When should you use it?

It is very beneficial for the liver because it increases bile production (choleretic) and facilitates emptying of the gallbladder (cholagogue). So it is one of the most beneficial plants for liver disorders and gallbladder malfunction. It also has the ability to stimulate the appetite, aid digestion, and exert a mild laxative effect for preventing constipation. Used orally as herbal tea, fresh salad, or two or three tablespoons of fresh juice before meals, it has a diuretic and cleansing effect, which is highly recommended for preventing water retention and for removing calcium oxalate crystals to prevent kidney stones. This, together with its important work in supporting the liver, makes it an effective treatment against eczema, rashes, and boils, which are often caused by autointoxication. Dandelion is often recommended when seasons are changing. It is an effective treatment for overeating, which makes it useful for weight control.

Moreover, applying it externally as a poultice helps heal wounds and bruises.

Presentation

Its freshly picked leaves can be used to prepare a fresh juice, using a blender, and then added to a salad. If you cannot get it fresh, it is available as troches (dried and ground) or in teabags, ready for preparing infusions and decoctions; it also comes in (½ to 1 teaspoon [2 to 5 milliliters] every 8 hours), liquid extract (¾ to 2 teaspoons [4 to 10 milliliters] every 8 hours), and capsules (powdered or dry).

Remedies

By itself

Digestive and cleansing infusion: add a teaspoon of dandelion to a cup of boiling water. Let it steep for 10 minutes and strain. Drink 3 cups a day, half an hour before meals. This remedy not only helps with digestion, but it cleanses the entire body.

Combined

Hepatoprotective and diuretic infusion: mix equal parts boldo, artichoke, dandelion, and peppermint. Add a teaspoon of this mixture to a cup of boiling water and let it steep for 10 minutes. Strain it and drink it before meals. It will help good digestion and facilitate excretion of waste substances.

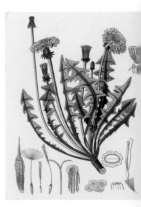

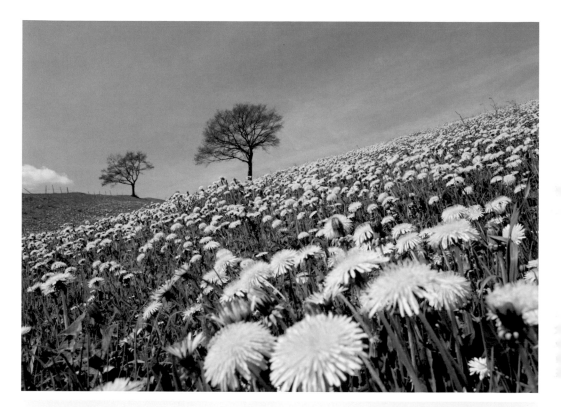

Precautions
Do not use during pregnancy or lactation, for young children, or persons suffering from bile duct obstruction. If you have gallstones, consult with a specialist before using it.

Description
It grows to about 1 foot (30 centimeters) high, and its toothed or lobed leaves form a rosette at ground level. Its stems have yellow flowers, which mature into white blowballs that can be spread over long distances by simply blowing on them.

Cultivation
It is very common in meadows, fields and roadsides across Europe and America.

Harvesting
For medicinal purposes, its leaves are harvested in spring, and its roots are harvested in fall or late summer. To preserve it, the useful parts are dried and stored in a sealed opaque glass container, away from moisture.

Composition
Some of its active components include lactones, triterpenes, steroids, phenolic acids, carotenoids, minerals, and polysaccharides such as inulin and mucilage.

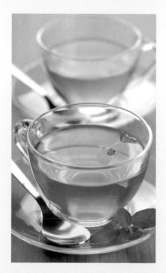

Fumitory

(Fumaria officinalis)

Clears the liver and purifies the body

The word "fumitory" comes from the Latin *fumus* ("smoke"), although it is not known whether it is because when it is crushed it makes you cry just as smoke does, or because its leaves resemble the smoke from a fire. In fact, old sorcerers believed that when this plant was set on fire, its smoke would drive away evil spirits.

When should you use it?

It has antispasmodic, diuretic, and cleansing properties, but what stands out most is its ability to promote smooth gallbladder function, from its cholagogue and choleretic effect, significantly improving the digestive process. Fumitory is recommended to relieve heavy and difficult digestions, migraines, and intestinal spasms.

Used externally, it is a good emollient for relieving eczema and rashes.

Presentation

Collect it in the wild, then dry it in the shade, and keep in tightly closed glass containers, away from light. You can find it in troches (dried and ground), ready for making tea. It is also possible to buy it as fluid or dry extract and in capsules, the latter being the most practical because its dosage, indications, and expiration date are specified by the manufacturer.

Remedies

BY ITSELF

Digestive infusion: add 1 teaspoon of fumitory to a cup of boiling water. Let it steep for 10 minutes and strain. You can sweeten it with honey or sugar, and then drink 3 cups a day before meals.

COMBINED

Herbal tea for gallstones: mix equal parts boldo, dandelion, peppermint, and fumitory. Place a teaspoon of this mixture into a cup and add boiling water. Let it steep for 10 minutes and strain. Drink 3 cups a day to digest fats and remove toxins, for treating gallstones.

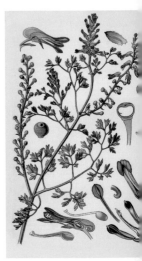

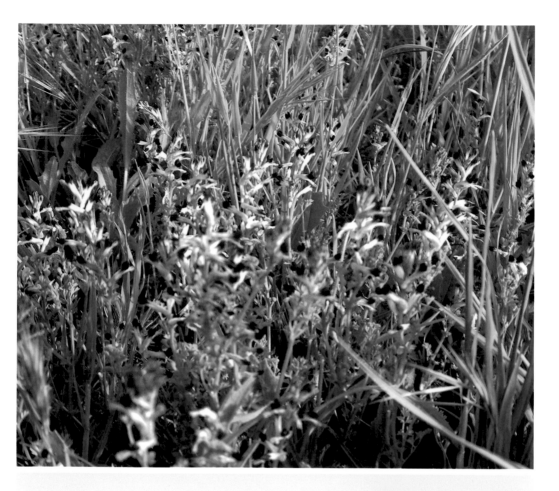

Precautions
Fumitory should not be administered to pregnant or nursing women, young children, or those suffering from bile duct obstruction. If you are suffering from gallstones, consult with a specialist before using.

Description
It is an herbaceous annual plant, which grows to 7.8 to 27 inches (20 to 70 centimeters) high. Its leaves are gray-green, and its flowers are pink or red. It smells sour and tastes bitter.

Cultivation
It is common near farm fields, on roadsides, and in vacant lots. It is native to Europe, but it has spread throughout the world.

Harvesting
The entire fumitory plant is used, except the root. It can be collected in the spring, from April to June.

Composition
It contains alkaloids, flavonoids, mucilage, tannins, organic acids, and minerals, among other things.

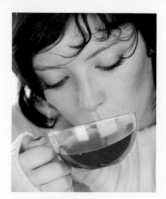

Birch

(Betula pendula)

Ally for kidney health

It has always been recognized and appreciated for its diuretic virtues, and although it has a delicate appearance, its thin and flexible rods were once used for birching. Its wood and coal are of very good quality, and shepherds used its waterproof bark to make tumblers.

When should you use it?

Since it contains flavonoids, it has a valuable diuretic effect, but unlike other diuretics, birch does not cause loss of large amounts of minerals, nor does it irritate kidney tissue, but rather it has the ability to reduce inflammation and regenerate kidney tissue. It is often used to "rinse out" the urinary tract as a treatment for genitourinary infections because it increases urination, which eliminates pathogens. It is also used effectively for preventing lithiasis in the kidneys and bladder, because it helps to eliminate calcium oxalate microcrystals. Indeed, in some cases, it can even eliminate existent calculi. This same diuretic property is used as a supplement in the treatment of rheumatic diseases and gout, for weight loss, and for cleansing and detoxifying.

Moreover, it increases bile secretion (cholagogue), which helps digestion and lowers high cholesterol levels (lipid lowering).

Externally, birch bark is rich in tannins, which give it an astringent and antiseptic effect for healing wounds.

Presentation

It is very common to drink it as a tea (1 or 2 teaspoons per cup) that is prepared with dried leaves and chopped birch. It is also commonly used in capsules or tablets and liquid extract (½ to 1 teaspoon [3 to 5 grams] per day, divided into 3 doses). And it is part of many diuretic and cleansing mixtures, usually for infusions, but also in tablets and capsules.

Remedies

BY ITSELF

Purifying tea: add a tablespoon of birch leaves to a cup of boiling water. Let it steep for 10 minutes and strain. It can be sweetened with honey or sugar. Drink 2 or 3 cups a day.

COMBINED

Diuretic herbal tea: Mix equal parts birch leaves, corn stigmas, and goldenrod flowers. Add a tablespoon of this mixture to a cup of boiling water. Let it steep for 10 minutes and strain. Drink 3 cups a day to treat water retention, eliminate waste substances, and prevent kidney stones.

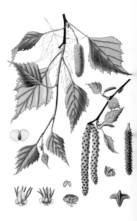

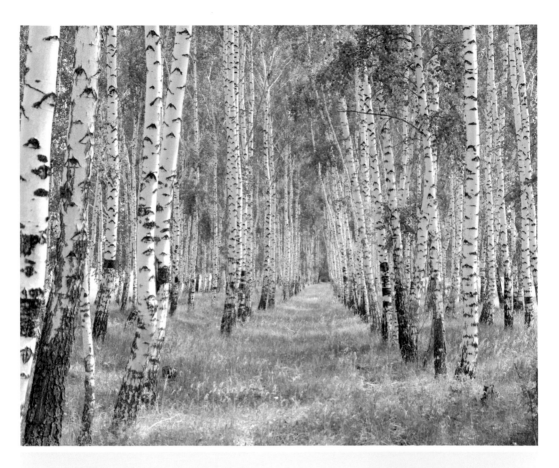

Precautions

It is contraindicated for persons suffering from peptic ulcer and gastritis. It is also not recommended during pregnancy and lactation. If you suffer from kidney or heart failure, consult with a specialist before using.

Description

It is a large tree (reaching up to 98 feet [30 meters]) with a round and irregular treetop. Young branches have white-silver bark. Its heart-shaped leaves are stalked at the base. Its unisexual flowers grow together in yellowish green catkins.

Cultivation

It is grown in gardens, in cold-temperate regions in the northern hemisphere, and cleared forest areas.

Harvesting

Its leaves and sometimes its bark are used.

Composition

Its leaves are rich in triterpene, saponins, flavonoids, phenolic acids, and vitamin C. Its bark contains tannin, essential oils, and diterpenes.

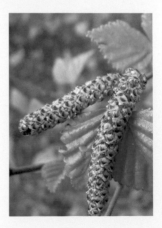

Heather

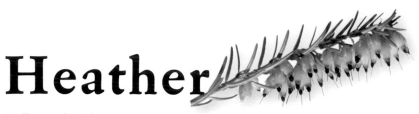

(Calluna vulgaris)

Enemy of urinary tract infections

Bees prefer it for making honey. In late summer, its green color and purple flowers cover meadows and sandy soils.

When should you use it?

It is a good remedy against genitourinary infections. This is because it works as a urinary antiseptic with a powerful antibacterial effect, which is strengthened by its diuretic action. By increasing urine output, it also eliminates germs that are responsible for these disorders. Although it is not often used to prevent edema (fluid retention) and kidney stones, it could reasonably be used as treatments for either. Its astringent properties help to stop diarrhea.

Presentation

Its flower tops are dried and chopped for making tea (1 or 2 teaspoons per cup), and they are available in capsule form, with micronized powder. You can also find it in liquid extract (¼ to ¾ teaspoon (1.5 to 3 milliliters) every 8 hours) and tinctures. Externally, it can be used for baths (1 cup per quart (250 grams per liter) of water).

Remedies

BY ITSELF

Infusion for urinary tract infection: add a teaspoon of heather to a cup of boiling water and let it steep for 10 minutes. Strain and sweeten with honey or sugar, if desired. Drink 1 cup every 6 hours, preferably after meals. Do not continue treatment for longer than 1 week.

COMBINED

To reinforce its effect, heather is usually combined with other antiseptic and diuretic plants such as bearberry and Java tea.

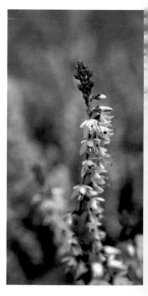

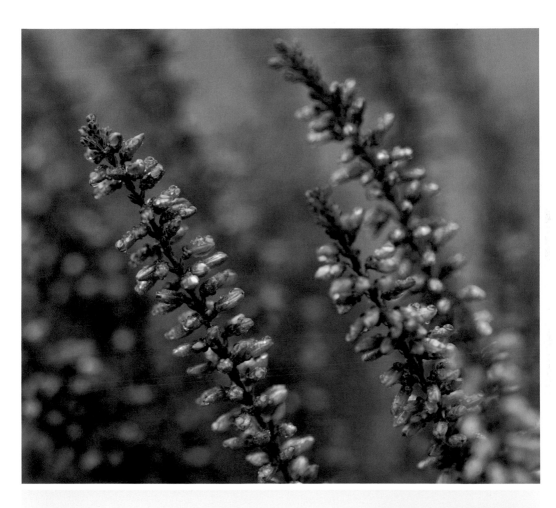

Precautions
It is contraindicated during pregnancy and lactation, and for children under the age of 12. For liver, kidney, or heart failure, consult with a specialist before using it.

Description
It is a dwarf and winding bush. Its many branches are thin and covered with small and persistent lanceolate leaves. Its pink flowers grow in clusters.

Cultivation
This bush grows in siliceous soils in the northern hemisphere.

Harvesting
Its flowering tops are harvested when they begin to bloom.

Composition
It is rich in simple phenols, glycosides (like arbutin), tannins, flavonoids, triterpenes, phenolic compounds, and steroids.

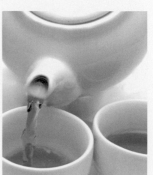

Bearberry

(Arctostaphylos uva-ursi)

Powerful urinary antiseptic

Since ancient times, in Scandinavia and the British Isles, bearberry was used as a medicinal plant. However, in Greece and Rome it was not known. Its use became more widespread, and in the 18th century, its medicinal virtues for urinary disorders became known throughout Europe and America.

When should you use it?

It has a strong antibiotic and antiseptic effect on the urinary organs. It also has diuretic and anti-inflammatory activity. So it is easy to see why it is an excellent remedy for treating all kinds of urinary tract infections, such as chronic cystitis, prostatitis, and urethritis. Maintain a diet rich in fruit and vegetables such as tomatoes, or try using bicarbonate (½ to 1 teaspoon [6 to 8 grams] a day) to maintain the alkaline pH level of urine and thus reinforce the effects of bearberry.

It is also very effective for preventing kidney stones; some even say that it can dissolve them. This latter claim has not been demonstrated, but in any case, it is beneficial for these conditions because it prevents urine infection that is typical of these disorders.

Bearberry gives urine a greenish color, indicating that treatment is proving effective.

Presentation

It is typically used dried and chopped, ready for preparing tea (½ teaspoon [3 grams] per cup every 6 hours) or in the form of capsules containing powdered dry leaves. Although less frequent, it can be purchased in the form of liquid extract (½ to ¾ teaspoon [2 to 3 milliliters] once a day) and as an ingredient in mixtures for infusion with other diuretic and antiseptic plants.

Remedies

BY ITSELF

Decoction for cystitis: use ½ to 2 tablespoons (10 to 30 grams)of bearberry per quart (liter) of water. Let it steep for 3 or 4 hours and then boil it for 15 minutes. Strain it and drink a cup every 3 or 4 hours, up to 4 cups (1 liter) a day. Do not use bearberry as a treatment for longer than a week or more than 5 times a year without a prescription.

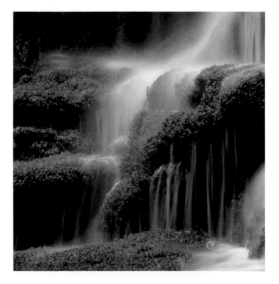

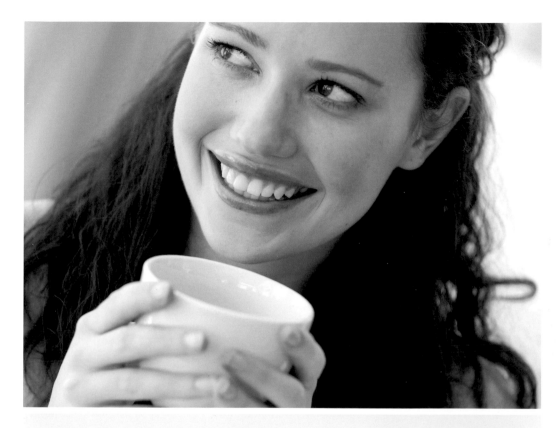

Precautions

Avoid ingesting bearberry during pregnancy and lactation, or if you suffer from peptic ulcer, and do not administer it to children under the age of 12. Persons with renal failure, liver failure, or heart failure must use it with caution.

Description

It is a woody shrub that grows 5 to 11 inches (15 to 30 centimeters) high. Its stems are long and crawling, and its perennials leaves are small and dark green. Its white or pink flowers are round, and its fruit is a round, bright red berry.

Cultivation

Although it is native to northern Europe and Asia, today it is widespread throughout Europe and North America. It grows abundantly in soils that are rich in silica and on mountainsides.

Harvesting

Its leaves are collected throughout the year, preferably in the summer. They are dried with hot air and stored in tightly sealed containers, away from light and moisture.

Composition

It contains phenols, phenolic acids, tannins, iridoids, flavonoids, and triterpenes.

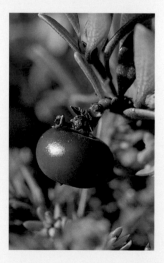

Corn

(Zea mays)

Soft but powerful diuretic

Besides being a staple food for pre-Columbian natives, corn kernels have been used for medicinal purposes since ancient times. Currently, it remains a staple food for many people, but for its therapeutic properties, we use its styles or stigmas we call silk.

When should you use it?

It is noted for its ability to increase urination, as well as its antispasmodic and anti-inflammatory effect on the urinary tract. It is a very well tolerated remedy that does not irritate the kidneys and does not cause electrolyte imbalance in the blood. It is recommended for the prevention and treatment of kidney stones, because by increasing urine output, it expels out calcium oxalate microcrystals. It also plays an important role against urinary tract infection because it helps remove pathogenic microorganisms. It also works well as a remedy for fluid retention, swollen legs, and hypertension.

For external use, thanks to its allantoin content, it can heal scratches and other minor injuries.

Presentation

The most common way to use it is in the form of infusions (1 tablespoon per quart [10 grams per liter] of water, drink a cup several times a day) and capsules containing dry extract. It can also be used in liquid extract (¼ to ½ teaspoon [1.5 to 2.5 milliliters] every 6 hours) and tincture (½ to 1 teaspoon [2.5 to 5 milliliters] every 6 hours).

Remedies

BY ITSELF

Diuretic infusion to prevent water retention: add a tablespoon of stigmas to a cup of boiling water and let it steep for 10 minutes, filter it, and drink it every 6 to 8 hours. This tea can be enjoyed hot or cold, morning or afternoon, but not at night.

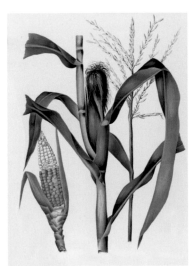

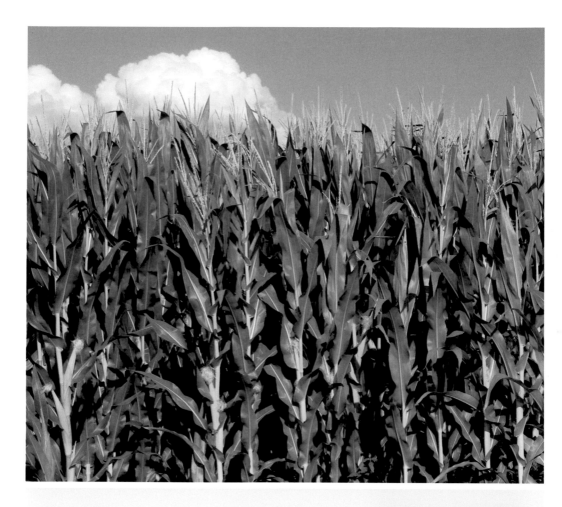

Precautions
If you suffer from heart or kidney failure, consult with a specialist before using it.

Description
It is an herbaceous plant of great size (3 to 10 feet [1 to 3 meters]), covered by broad, lanceolate, alternate leaves. Its male inflorescences are terminal spikes, while the female ones are large and surrounded by large bracts, from which numerous threadlike styles emerge.

Cultivation
It is native to South America, but it is cultivated worldwide.

Harvesting
Its styles are dried and kept in tightly closed containers away from light and humidity.

Composition
It contains minerals, flavonoids, saponins, tannins, steroids, allantoin, essential oil, and trace amounts of alkaloids.

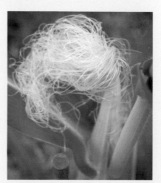

Aloe

(Aloe vera or A. barbadensis)

Great ally of health and beauty for your skin

A native to North Africa, aloe has been used since ancient times as traditional medicine by many civilizations. However, it was not until the end of World War II when its great efficacy as a therapeutic treatment was confirmed after it was used for burns.

When should you use it?

Applied externally, aloe gel stimulates skin regeneration, which accelerates wound healing and prevents infection and inflammation. It also has antiviral activity, so it can significantly improve herpes outbreaks. It also exerts radioprotective effect that prevents the skin from getting burned by ultraviolet radiation. Because of all these properties, aloe is one of the most complete and effective remedies for treating injuries, first and second-degree burns, sunburn, skin irritations, and abrasions. Similarly, it is highly recommended for psoriasis, eczema, acne, and fungal infections.

Due to its mucilage content, it also has moisturizing and softening properties that are used in cosmetics and other skin-care products.

Moreover, it is purifying and toning when it is ingested orally. It is used as a digestive for treating peptic ulcer.

Presentation

You can find fresh aloe juice, but it is still most commonly available in gel form where it is the main ingredient (usually contains 10 to 70 percent aloe), or in many products that combine aloe with other ingredients (moisturizers, sunscreens, after-sun products, shower gels, shaving creams, face masks, lipsticks, etc.).

You can also obtain pure aloe gel at home. Just have it planted in pots or in the garden and cut a leaf into 2-inch (5-centimeter) pieces, then slice these smaller pieces and let them drain. Store its gel in a tightly closed glass jar, away from light, heat, and moisture.

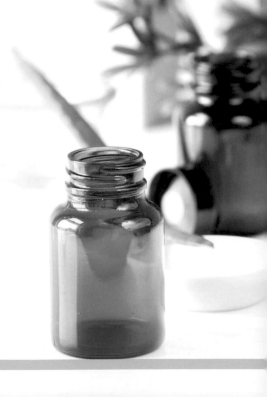

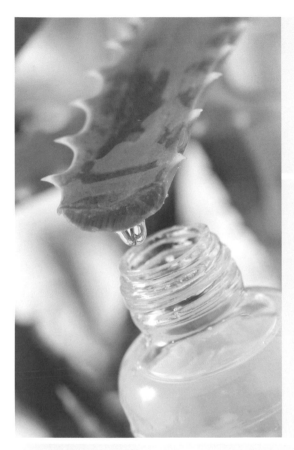

Aloe juice

Aloe gel is sticky, transparent, and tasteless and should not be confused with aloe juice. Although they are obtained from the same leaves, they are very different. The gel is used topically as treatment for burns and skin irritations. Its juice is mainly used as a laxative.

Curiosities

● There are over 350 species of aloe, but only a few have therapeutic applications; the most prominent are Aloe barbadensis Miller (or Aloe vera L.), known as Barbados aloe, and Aloe ferox Miller also called Cape aloe.
● Aloe has been used as traditional medicine by many civilizations since ancient times. The Chinese were the first to use it. It was often used in ancient Egypt. Historical Roman, Greek, Hindu, and Arab documents describe its medicinal and cosmetic virtues. The Spaniards brought it with them to America during their conquest and introduced it to the plantations of the West Indies and the semi-warm regions of the southern United States.

● **Precautions**
It should not be used orally during pregnancy and lactation, or for children under six.

● **Description**
It looks like a cactus but it is actually a perennial plant that is characterized by its green, elongated, hard, and fleshy leaves that usually have thorns along their edges. Its yellow or red flowers, depending on the variety, grow on a long stem.

● **Cultivation**
It is native to southern Africa, but it has spread to warm desert regions of America and Asia. In Spain, it grows in the south of the peninsula and the Canary Islands. It grows in dry and sunny environments with low rainfall.

● **Harvesting**
Primarily, the gel or juice is used after it is obtained from the fleshy pulp of its leaves. It can be collected at any time.

● **Composition**
It contains mostly water and abundant polysaccharides, amino acids, enzymes, mineral salts, and vitamins.

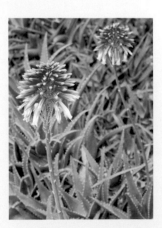

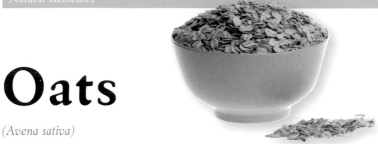

Oats

(Avena sativa)

Moisturizes and soothes dry skin

For centuries, it has been the staple food of people known for their strength, such as the Scots, who considered it a symbol of strength. Not surprisingly, it is a cereal with high energy and nutritional value, but it is also medicinal. It is used to calm the nerves, and it is one of the main ingredients in many cosmetics that are used for daily skin care.

When should you use it?

Applied externally, it is used for its emollient and regenerative properties. It moisturizes, softens, and protects all skin types, even baby skin, and especially, dry, sensitive, or irritated skin. These properties are attributed to its richness in silicon and mucilage. Taken orally, it is good for balancing the nervous system because it can both relax and strengthen. Its relaxing effect is due to the fact that it contains small amounts of nontoxic alkaloid, avenin, which gives it a sedative effect. It is used as a sleeping aid for insomnia. It can also be used as a supplement to reduce anxiety during a smoking cessation program. As for its strengthening effect, it is very effective in stimulating physical and mental capacity, and it is ideal for growing children, convalescents, athletes, or people who perform a lot of physical and intellectual activity.

Thanks to its mucilage, it also softens and protects intestinal mucosa, helping to improve digestion. It also helps to lower cholesterol and glucose.

Presentation

Most commonly, it is eaten like flakes with milk or yogurt, in muesli, or as an ingredient in other dishes. These same edible flakes and bran are used for making medicinal infusions. Also, it is used as an ingredient for sedatives and tonics and in cosmetics (bath gels and body creams for dry and sensitive skin).

Remedies

BY ITSELF

Oatmeal water: prepare a decoction by mixing 2 tablespoons of grains with 1 quart (liter) of water. Boil it for 5 minutes and then filter it. Sweeten it with honey and drink it throughout the day. It has a balancing and toning effect on the nervous system. Emollient bath: add this same decoction to your bath water to soften and moisturize the skin and relax the nerves.

COMBINED

Mix oatmeal, glycerin, and rose water to make a traditional anti-wrinkle ointment that works very well.

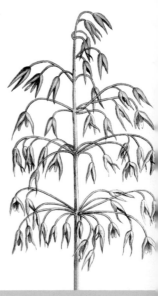

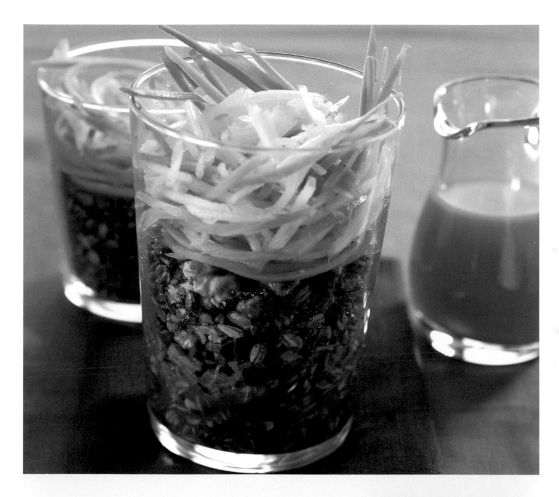

● **Precautions**

Oats are a cereal without any side effects whether ingested orally or applied externally to the skin.

● **Description**

It is an annual plant that grows up to 3 feet (1 meter) high, and its flowers, like its grains, are grouped in pairs, in spikes.

● **Cultivation**

Oats are native to southern Europe, but its cultivation has spread to the temperate regions throughout the world, especially in the northern hemisphere.

● **Harvesting**

Whole seeds (grains) and bran are used. It is sown in early spring, to be harvested in late summer.

● **Composition**

It is a source of polyunsaturated fatty acids (heart-healthy), vitamins, and minerals. It also contains phytosterols, enzymes, mucilage, and alkaloids (nontoxic).

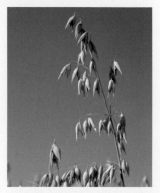

Burdock

(Arctium lappa)

Detoxifies and purifies the skin

This plant has existed for a long time, and its medicinal use has never been questioned. For therapeutic purposes, we use its root and leaves. It contains many active substances that exert a strong antibiotic and antiseptic effect especially on skin microorganisms. Not surprisingly, it used to be known as "ringworm grass," which perfectly illustrates its therapeutic usefulness.

When should you use it?

Stimulates emptying of bile from the gallbladder to the intestine (cholagogue effect), it has sudorific and diuretic activity. For all this, it is easy to understand that burdock has an important purifying role in facilitating the elimination of toxins through both urine and through the skin. This, together with its strong antimicrobial and antifungal effect, makes burdock a particularly effective remedy against bacteria that cause skin infections, and as treatment for acne and oily skin. It is also useful for chronic eczema and other skin infections such as abscesses or infected cysts, as well as recurrent urinary tract infections such as cystitis.

It works best when it is simultaneously applied topically and ingested orally.

Presentation

The most common way to use it is in troches (dried and ground) for infusions and decoctions (3 tablespoons per quart [40 grams per liter]) mouth-washes (gargling), liniments, compresses, and other preparations. You can also purchase it in liquid extract (¼ to ½ teaspoon [1 to 2.5 milliliters] every 8 hours) and tincture (½ to 1 teaspoon [2.5 to 5 milliliters] every 8 hours), or in capsules. It is also an ingredient in numerous preparations for external use, such as creams and gels.

Remedies

BY ITSELF

Purifying herbal tea: mix a teaspoon of burdock root per cup of water. Boil for about 10 minutes and let it steep for 5 minutes. Strain it and sweeten it with honey or sugar, if you like. Drink a cup every 8 hours, throughout the duration of the infection. To enhance its effect, use this decoction to apply compresses on the affected area for 15 minutes twice a day.

COMBINED

Herbal tea for acne: mix equal parts nettle, pansy, and burdock root. Add a teaspoon of this mixture to a cup of boiling water and let it steep for 10 minutes. Strain it and drink a cup every 8 hours. It helps eliminate toxins that worsen skin condition.

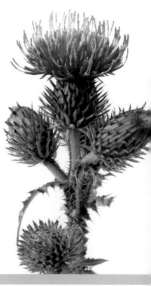

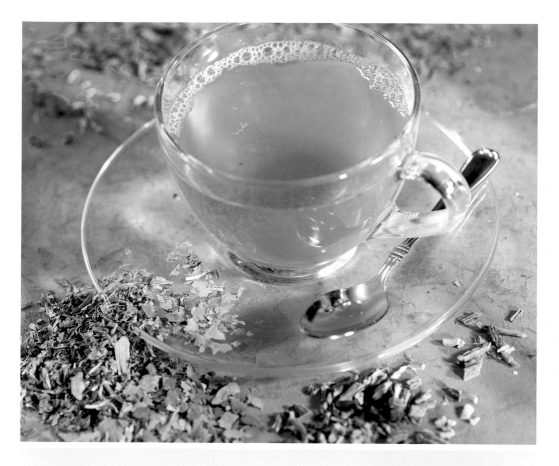

● **Precautions**
For oral use, it is not recommended during pregnancy and lactation.

● **Description**
It is a herbaceous and robust plant that grows over 3 feet (1 meter) high. Its large leaves are coated with fuzz on the underside. Its flowers are purplish florets.

● **Cultivation**
It is abundant near inhabited areas, roads, and landfills in temperate regions of Europe and America, although it is best not to collect it in such places as they may be polluted.

● **Harvesting**
Its root and leaves are used. You must wait for the spring of the second year of cultivation to harvest its root. Once collected, rinse it with water, cut it into pieces, and dry it as soon as possible in the shade and in a well-ventilated area. Store it in a tightly sealed glass jar.

● **Composition**
It contains lactones (arctiopicrina), triterpenoids, inulin, mucilage, phenolic acids, tannins, and essential oil.

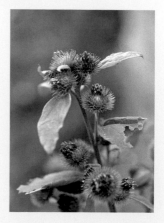

Borage

(Borago officinalis)

Prevents wrinkles

Great ally of the beauty of the skin, it is a common ingredient in cleansing and detoxifying cures. Its name seems to be of Arab origin: *abu rash*, which means "father of sweat," referring to the strong sudorific property of its flowers. In addition to its numerous medicinal and cosmetic virtues, it is prized for its culinary uses, which are well known.

When should you use it?

Its diuretic and sudorific effect make borage an excellent blood purifier, and it helps to eliminate toxins from the body through urine and sweat. Its abundance of mucilage, a type of emollient fiber, not only produces a slight beneficial laxative effect for constipation, but ingesting it is beneficial for gastric disorders as well as colds because it softens mucus and facilitates expectoration.

For external use, it is soothing and anti-inflammatory, so it is a good remedy to improve the appearance of the skin if you suffer from dermatitis or eczema.

Borage oil is an ideal choice to combat skin dryness and lack of elasticity that cause the first wrinkles. Borage oil is extracted from the seeds, and it is very rich in unsaturated essential fatty acids.

Take two or four capsules of this oil a day, to moisturize and nourish the skin from within, fortifying and toning deep wrinkles that may already be in place. It also helps to normalize menstrual cycles, with its hormone-balancing properties, so it is very useful for PMS.

Presentation

One of the most common ways to consume it is fresh in salad. You can also buy it dried and chopped ready for making infusions (2 teaspoons per quart [10 grams per liter]) and in liquid extract (¼ teaspoon [0.5 to 1.5 milliliters] every 8 hours). Oil capsules can be taken orally or applied topically. It is an ingredient in topical creams and gels.

Remedies

BY ITSELF
Purifying herbal tea: add a teaspoon of borage to a cup of boiling water. Let it steep for 10 minutes and strain. Drink 3 cups a day, but remember not to use it for an extended period of time.

You can use this same infusion and apply it externally as plasters to moisturize and soften the skin. Alternatively, use a few quarts (liters) of this same infusion in your bath water.

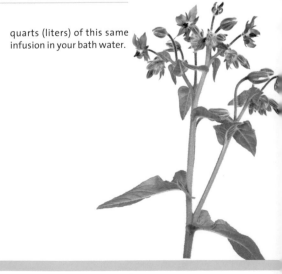

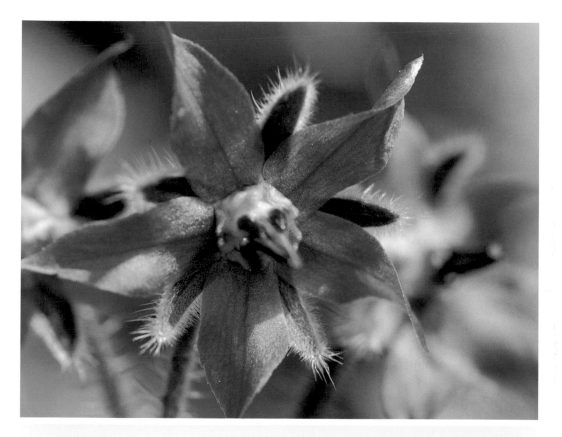

● Precautions

It is not recommended for oral use during pregnancy or lactation, or for persons suffering from liver failure.

● Description

It is a herbaceous plant that grows 1 to 2.3 feet (30 to 70 centimeters) high. It is easily recognizable by the hairs that cover its stems and leaves, but especially by its showy blue flowers.

● Cultivation

It is native to the Mediterranean area and grows wild in moist, fertile soil, on roadsides, and in sandy soils that get a lot of sun.

● Harvesting

Its flowers, leaves, and stems are used. The best time to harvest them is in the spring. Dry them as soon as possible in a shaded and well-ventilated area. Store them in tightly closed glass jars. Its oil is extracted by cold pressing its seeds.

● Composition

It contains oil (rich in unsaturated fatty acids), mucilage, mineral salts, alkaloids, tannins, saponins, and flavonoids.

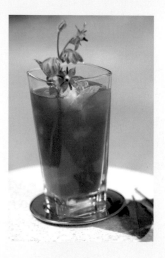

Marigold

(Calendula officinalis)

Pampers and protects the skin

It is not clear where it came from, but it is supposed to be native to the Mediterranean, where it grows spontaneously. It is often found in gardens and planters for their colorful beauty, and for centuries it has been used as a medicinal plant. Currently, it is considered a very valuable remedy that is devoid of toxicity, for use in skin care.

When should you use it

Applied externally, it is healing, as it can accelerate re-epithelialization of damaged skin by stimulating collagen synthesis. It also has an anti-inflammatory, antiseptic, and calming effect. It is one of the most common and effective treatments for superficial skin wounds, such as cuts and scrapes, helping to make the wound heal faster. It is also used to treat eczema, dermatitis, and burns. Even gargling with an infusion of marigold may relieve inflammation and sore throat, stomatitis, and pharyngitis. This plant has an emollient effect, which smooths, tones, and moisturizes the skin, and protects and beautifies dry and sensitive skin. It is very good for repairing cracked skin of the hands. It also calms and clears sunburned skin; that is why it is often found in the ingredient list of many creams and gels recommended for after sunbathing. It is also a good remedy for reducing inflammation and itching caused by insect bites.

Presentation

For external use, this plant is very popular. It is available dried and ground, in bags without any indicated dosage for preparing teas and homemade maceration, in tinctures (1 to 2 teaspoons [5 to 10 milliliters] several applications a day), and liquid extracts (¼ to ½ teaspoon [1 to 2 milliliters] in various applications a day). In addition, there are many preparations that have marigold as their main ingredient, such as oils, sun lotions, ointments, creams, and shampoos.

Remedies

BY ITSELF

Infusion of marigold: add a teaspoon of flowers to a cup of boiling water. Let it steep for 10 minutes and strain. Once it is warm, use it to apply as compresses or for gargling to relieve mouth and throat infections.

Marigold oil: This is one of the most popular home remedies for burns. Macerate a handful of flowers in a quart (liter) of virgin olive oil for about 40 days in a warm place away from direct sunlight.

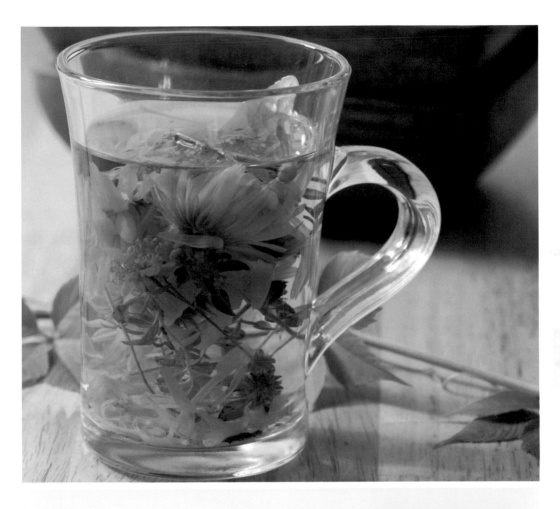

● Precautions

For external use, there are no contraindications except if you are allergic to it.

● Description

It is a very showy herbaceous plant whose yellow flowers close at night and open at dawn. The flowering period lasts almost all year. It can measure 11 to 20 inches (30 to 50 centimeters) high, and its leaves are alternate, fleshy, and long.

● Cultivation

It is grown in European and American gardens, although it can also be found wild, near villages, in meadows, roadsides, and orchards.

● Harvesting

Its flowers are harvested from June to September.

● Composition

It contains saponins, triterpenes, flavonoids, carotenoids, mucilage, and essential oil.

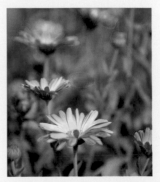

Sarsaparilla

(Smilax sarsaparilla)

Acne enemy

It was known by Dioscorides and its popularity peaked when, in the 17th century, the Spaniards named many American species of the same genus as sarsaparilla, and believed they had found a cure for syphilis. Today, we know for sure that the root of this plant has purifying properties that can relieve some skin problems, and we can still use it to make "sarsaparilla," which is an old but very refreshing drink.

When should you use it?

It has diuretic and sudorific properties, but what stands out is its purifying power, which facilitates the elimination of toxins through urine. In this sense, it works very well when combined with other purifying plants that enhance its effects. It has stimulating and strengthening properties so it has traditionally been used as a digestive and expectorant remedy to treat bronchitis. Applied externally, it removes impurities effectively so it clears up acne and other skin conditions such as eczema and psoriasis.

Presentation

Its roots are available dried and crushed, ready for making decoctions and tea (1 teaspoon per cup), in fluid extract (¼ to 1 teaspoon [1 to 5 milliliters] every 24 hours), and tincture (1 to 3 teaspoons [5 to 15 milliliters] once a day). If you prefer, take it in capsules filled with root powder (dosage is indicated by the manufacturer) or in mixtures for preparing cleanses, in which sarsaparilla is combined with other diuretic plants.

Remedies

BY ITSELF

Purifying herbal tea: mix a teaspoon of the root per cup of water. Boil it for 10 minutes and let it steep for 5 minutes. Strain it and if you like, you can sweeten it with honey or sugar. This infusion will help eliminate toxins. Drink up to 3 cups a day.

COMBINED

To visibly improve your skin, prepare an infusion by mixing equal parts sarsaparilla, burdock, dandelion, and corn silk and drink it in small portions throughout the day; or mix equal parts sarsaparilla, nettle, fumitory, horsetail, and walnut leaves and drink 2 cups a day.

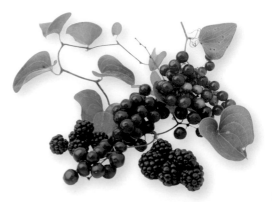

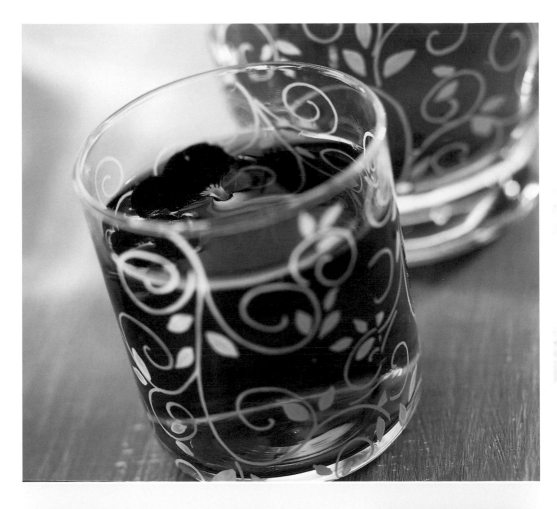

Precautions
Avoid using sarsaparilla in high doses and for prolonged treatment. Consult with your doctor if you want to use it as a diuretic but you are suffering from hypertension or kidney failure.

Description
It is a thorny shrub that climbs trees up to 49 feet (15 meters) feet (15 meters) high. Its heart-shaped leaves are large and lined with thorns. The flowers are white and the fruits are red or blackish.

Cultivation
The European species is very common in forests and hedgerows, although American sarsaparilla is much more appreciated for herbal medicine.

Harvesting
Its root is collected in spring or autumn.

Composition
Other components include saponins and minerals.

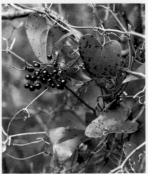

Garlic

(Allium sativum)

Allied against infections

It adds a very Mediterranean flavor to culinary creations, and its medicinal virtues were well-known to the ancient Egyptians, Hebrews, Greeks, and Romans. It is the main ingredient in many dishes, to which it gives its aroma and flavor, as well as its beneficial properties. Its volatile sulfur compounds are the reason for its properties and scent.

When should you use it?

You could say that garlic is a "cure-all" because it has many health benefits. It is known for its excellent diuretic, cleansing, antiseptic, and antibiotic properties, along with its ability to enhance the body's defenses, which make it a very effective treatment for respiratory infections like bronchitis and colds, and for curing urinary tract infections. It also works as a vasodilator to thin the blood (anti-coagulant), which promotes blood circulation and prevents blood clots. It also lowers blood pressure and high cholesterol and, last but not least, it is a powerful antioxidant.

Applied externally, it effectively removes corns and warts.

Raw garlic is not well liked because it leaves us with bad breath, but it is more effective than cooked garlic. To get the most out of it, include it in your diet every day, which you can easily do since it is a very versatile ingredient. Only those with delicate stomachs may find it indigestible.

Presentation

It is easily available to everyone because all you need is one or two cloves of garlic a day. You can also find it as essential oil, or in capsules (with garlic powder) that are very practical and easy to use if you hate garlic breath.

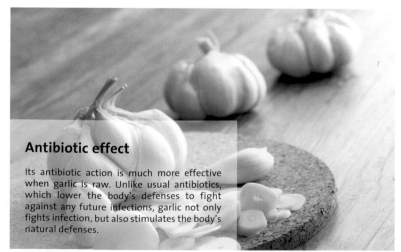

Antibiotic effect

Its antibiotic action is much more effective when garlic is raw. Unlike usual antibiotics, which lower the body's defenses to fight against any future infections, garlic not only fights infection, but also stimulates the body's natural defenses.

Curiosities

The Greeks regarded garlic as a source of physical strength, and therefore they offered it to athletes before competitions at the Olympic games. In Egypt, garlic was planted at crossroads as a sign of protection against curses. In the Middle Ages it was used against the plague, and physicians applied garlic masks on those affected by the plague.

Its smell is not very strong when the bulbs are intact, but when it is cut or crushed, it immediately releases its intense smell due to the formation of volatile sulfur compounds (alliin, allyl disulfide, etc.), to which we can attribute its beneficial effects.

Precautions
It is not recommended for use during breastfeeding, and people with blood-clotting disorders have to use it very carefully.

Description
It is a herbaceous bulbous plant with an erect or curved stem and broad flat leaves. Its white or reddish flowers grow clustered together in umbels. The bulb is made up of about 10 to 12 cloves.

Cultivation
Garlic is native to Central Asia, but its cultivation has spread throughout the world. It is grown in sunny gardens.

Harvesting
Its bulb is harvested from June to July, placed on the ground to dry in the sun for 2 to 3 days, then hung on strings and stored in a well-ventilated place.

Composition
It contains sulfoxide, homogeneous polysaccharides, saponins, and mineral salts.

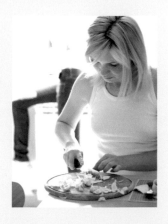

Siberian ginseng

(Eleutherococcus senticosus)

Combats physical and mental fatigue

This plant is very abundant in Siberia, where it is also known as "Russian secret plant" because when its extraordinary virtues were discovered, they were kept secret for a long time. After it was finally introduced to modern herbal medicine, and its ability to fight fatigue was thoroughly demonstrated, its importance increased.

When should you use it?

Fresh or dried, it is an extraordinary remedy against physical or mental exhaustion, stress, depression, and convalescence because it is a good restorative remedy that helps invigorate the nervous system by replenishing energy. It increases physical performance in athletes, reduces fatigue, and is recommended as a sexual stimulant. It also increases concentration and memory, so it is very good for students studying for exams and for persons who do a lot of mental work. It boosts the body's natural defenses against bacterial and viral infections, increases blood hemoglobin levels thus preventing anemia, and decreases blood glucose levels, which is very beneficial for people with diabetes.

Presentation

It is most often available in capsules with powder or dried root extract, and its recommended dosage is indicated by the manufacturer. You may also find its root, dried and ground, ready for making infusions (1 teaspoon per cup), in liquid extract (½ to ¾ teaspoon [2 to 3 milliliters] once a day), and tincture (2 teaspoons to 1 tablespoon [10 to 14 milliliters] once a day). Liquid extract and tincture are sold in opaque glass bottles to protect it from light. It can be purchased in ampoules, alone or combined with other plants.

Remedies

BY ITSELF
Usually, it is taken in capsules or tablets with a glass of water. The recommended amounts are ½ teaspoon (2 or 3 grams) per day, but the manufacturer will specify them. It is not advisable to use it for more than 3 consecutive months.

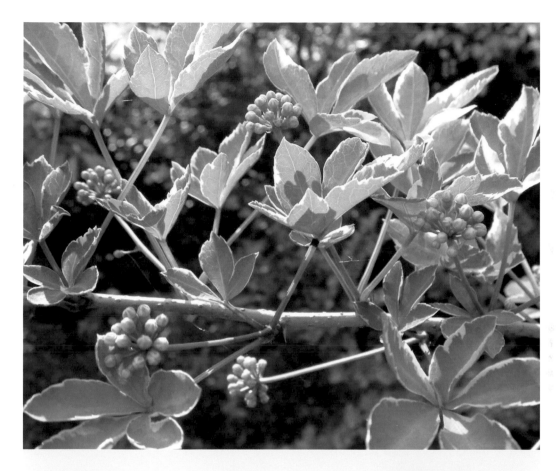

Precautions

It is contraindicated if you suffer from cardiac arrhythmias, hypertension, anxiety, nervousness, and during pregnancy and lactation. If you are being treated with digoxin, oral antidiabetic medication, or anticoagulants, you should consult with your doctor before using Siberian ginseng.

Description

It is a shrub that grows to 10 feet (3 meters) high. Its branches are covered with thorns, and its leaves grow in groups of five. Its flowers are grouped in bunches, and its fruit is a berry with five seeds.

Cultivation

It is native to the steppes of Siberia where it grows rampant and wild, in cedar forests and plains.

Harvesting

The roots and rhizomes are harvested at the end of spring or autumn.

Composition

Its most prominent active ingredients include eleutherosides, polysaccharides, and hydroxycoumarins.

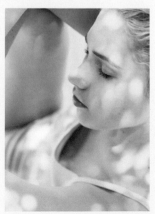

Echinacea

(Echinacea angustifolia)

The best protection against winter

Native Americans already knew its valuable properties and used it to treat snakebites and infected wounds, among other things. Until 1930, it was the best remedy for treating colds in the United States. Today, it is one of the best-researched and documented plants because of its important ability to prevent infections.

When should you use it?

It has a potent immunostimulant effect that can stimulate and strengthen the body's natural defenses, which significantly helps to tackle infectious diseases in general. It is particularly suitable for the prevention and treatment of respiratory infections, colds, and flu-like symptoms. It is a remedy that is highly recommended for those who are most vulnerable to disease, such as children, convalescents, and older adults. It is also used as a supplement to lessen the impact of side effects during cancer chemotherapy, because its powerful immunostimulatory action helps to eliminate toxins.

It is a good anti-inflammatory remedy that is applied externally to treat skin lesions such as wounds or burns. Its anti-infectious action helps heal and regenerate skin tissue.

Presentation

It is usually taken as tablets and capsules (dose is recommended by the manufacturer), liquid extract, syrup, and tincture (30 to 60 drops every 8 hours). You can buy its juice (1 to 2 tablespoons [6 to 9 milliliters] every 24 hours) extracted from parts of the plant that grow above ground. It is very commonly combined with other plants to fight the flu. Its use in troches (dried and chopped) for making tea is rare in our country. It is also an ingredient in healing ointments and creams.

Remedies

BY ITSELF

Herbal tea to boost your defenses: place a teaspoon of dried Echinacea in boiling water. Let it steep for 10 minutes and strain it. To relieve colds and boost your immune system, brew it fresh each day and drink 1 cup several times a day, hot and preferably between meals.

COMBINED

Herbal tea for colds: mix 1 part peppermint leaves, 1 part elderberries, 1 part hyssop, and ½ part of Echinacea. Add a teaspoon of this mixture to a cup of boiling water and let it steep for 10 minutes. Strain it and sweeten it with honey. Drink it freshly prepared and hot, 1 cup every 4 to 6 hours.

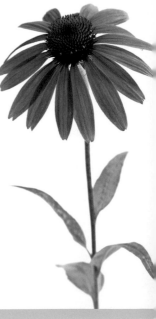

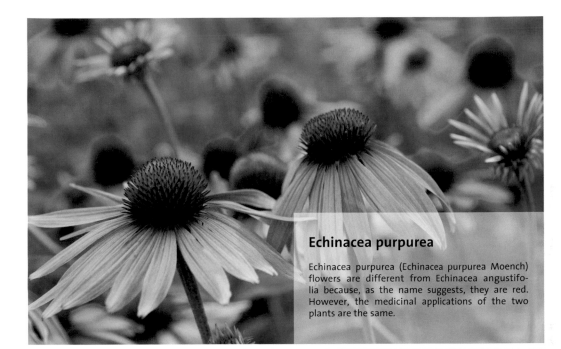

Echinacea purpurea

Echinacea purpurea (Echinacea purpurea Moench) flowers are different from Echinacea angustifolia because, as the name suggests, they are red. However, the medicinal applications of the two plants are the same.

Precautions
It not recommended for use during pregnancy and lactation. Echinacea may interact with certain drugs (such as corticosteroids, ketoconazole, etc.), so if you are taking any medication, it is best to consult with a specialist.

Description
It is a perennial plant that grows to 3 feet (1 meter) high. It has elongated, narrow, and rough leaves that are covered with hair. Its showy mauve flowers grow at the end of its stems.

Cultivation
It is native to North America and grows in the plains and sandy riverbanks of this continent. Currently, it is also grown for medicinal purposes in Central Europe.

Harvesting
Its root and parts of the plant that grow above ground are harvested in spring, after 4 years of cultivation. Once collected, they are dried in the shade, away from light and moisture.

Composition
Echinacea is notable for its content of heterogeneous polysaccharides, essential oil, phenolic acids, and polyyne.

Preventive treatment
Start taking echinacea 1 to 2 months before the beginning of winter (at low doses) to prevent infectious diseases, like colds and the flu. It is also a good prevention method when you are under physical or mental stress, which lowers and weakens your immune system.

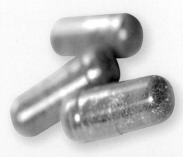

Buckthorn

(Hippophae rhamnoides)

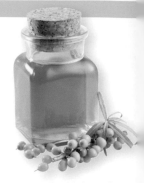

Revitalizes and strengthens the body

Since the 8th century, Tibetan pharmacopoeia already had preparations using buckthorn's berries. Although it is not well known in our country, it is very good for stimulating the body's defenses, and it is used as a nutritional supplement. This plant's oil is very rich in antioxidants and unsaturated fatty acids, so it is used in cosmetics.

When should you use it?

Because of its high vitamin C content, it has a strong overall toning effect, stimulates the body's defenses against infections, and helps you recover faster during convalescence. This makes it a good remedy to prevent influenza, coughing, colds, and fever.

It also strengthens and aids digestion because it is astringent and antidiarrheal. Furthermore, its berries are used as a nutritional supplement for those suffering from avitaminosis and overall weakness.

Furthermore, since its berries and oil are rich in unsaturated fatty acids and antioxidants, buckthorn can lower high cholesterol levels and prevent cardiovascular diseases. It fights premature aging and degenerative diseases.

Applied externally, its oil softens, moisturizes, and nourishes skin and slows signs of aging. It is good for recovering skin elasticity and smoothness because it stimulates cell regeneration. Its strong antioxidant action protects against solar radiation and cold, wind, and water. It is recommended for all skin types, especially dry or damaged skin.

Presentation

In our country, it is a fairly unknown remedy. It is very rarely used and is usually available as a nutritional supplement. Buckthorn jams made with its berries, juice, and some syrups are available in specialty stores. However, it is more frequently found as the main ingredient in creams or gels.

Remedies

By ITSELF

To stimulate the defenses and revitalize the body in general, eat three handfuls of ripe berries every day. The problem is that they are highly acidic and not everyone digests them well, so to make them easier to digest, you can prepare a homemade cough syrup. Extract the juice of ripe berries and boil it for 15 minutes, then add half its weight in sugar. Drink 3 tablespoons daily. It keeps well in a sealed container away from light.

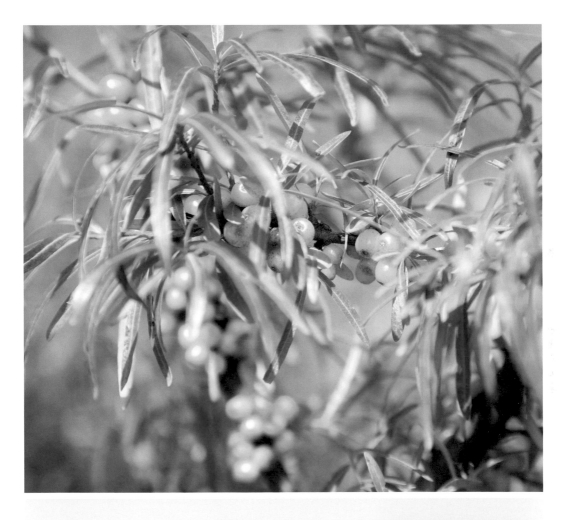

● **Precautions**
It has no toxicity.

● **Description**
It is a shrub that grows up to 16 feet (5 meters) high. Its branches are thorny, and its fruits are yellow or orange berries that are especially rich in vitamin C.

● **Harvesting**
Its berries and oil are used.

● **Composition**
Besides vitamin C, it contains carotenoids, vitamin E, unsaturated fatty acids such as oleic acid, flavonoids, phytosterols, mucilage, and tannins.

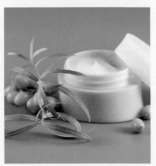

Ginseng

(Panax ginseng)

Natural stimulant

Prolonged stress and physical and mental fatigue can be overcome with the help of ginseng. Its root, which has a human shape, has been known for thousands of years in Chinese medicine as a stimulant and an aphrodisiac. Its generic name, *Panax*, derives from the Greek for "remedy for all illnesses," while "ginseng" comes from two Chinese words jin ("plant") and chen ("triad"), which refer to man, sky, and the plant.

When should you use it?

Ginseng is the best-known and -appreciated plant from the East. It improves mental acuity, sharpens memory, and increases concentration. Furthermore, it helps your body adapt to physically and mentally stressful situations, allowing it to vigorously confront any difficulties and prevent disease. It also increases physical resistance to cold, heat, and radiation.

It can work as a sexual stimulant because it can help men get and sustain an erection and help women feel sexually aroused. On the other hand, it has a slightly antidiabetic effect, which improves the efficiency of glucose, so it is useful for diabetics or those who are glucose intolerant. It also lowers blood cholesterol and triglycerides.

Presentation

Ginseng root is available in pieces, but it is better to use it in capsules or tablets with dosage amounts indicated by the manufacturer so as not to exceed the recommended dose.

Remedies

BY ITSELF

Invigorating: it is safer to take it in capsules or tablets and follow directions.

COMBINED

Stimulating solution: mix ginseng root powder with raw ginger juice and a little honey. Boil it and dissolve it in water. Drink this liquid up to 3 times a day.

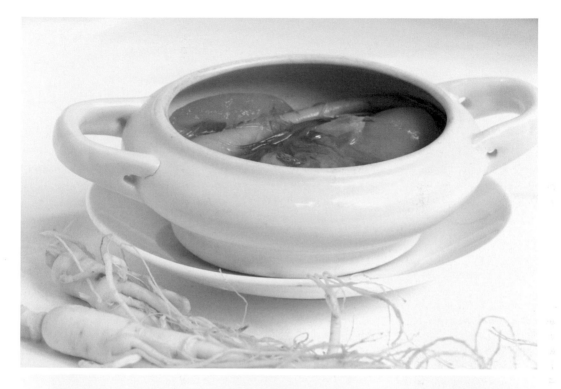

Precautions

Do not exceed the recommended dose (½ teaspoon [2 grams] at most per day), do not use it for an extended amount of time (never more than 3 months), and do not combine it with other stimulating substances, such as coffee or tea. Do not use it if you suffer from hypertension, tachycardia, insomnia, during pregnancy and lactation, or for children under the age of 12 because it can create anxiety and nervousness and raise blood pressure.

Description

Herbaceous plant that grows up to 3 feet (1 meter) high, with a spongy stem, oval leaves, and small purple or green flowers. Its whitish root is thick and fleshy, and ends in small fibrous roots.

Cultivation

The best-known ginseng is native to Korea, it is called red or Korean ginseng, and it contains more active ingredients. There is also Chinese ginseng, Russian or Siberian ginseng, Japanese ginseng, and American ginseng that is native to Wisconsin (United States).

Harvesting

Ginseng is grown in Korea, China, Japan, Bulgaria, and eastern Russia. In the fourth or fifth year of the plant, its root is collected, washed, and steamed before drying it. It is sliced and preserved.

Composition

It contains saponins, gingenosides, heterogeneous polysaccharides (panaxans), proteins, phenolic acids, polyyne, and steroids.

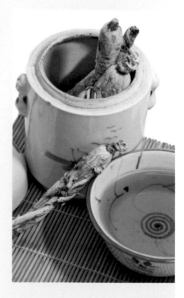

Cat's claw

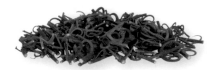

(Uncaria tomentosa)

Much more than a good anti-inflammatory

Since ancient times, it has been a very popular remedy among native people of the South American rainforest, where it is used to heal wounds, relieve muscle and joint pain, and even to treat women after childbirth. Today, there is great interest in its therapeutic effect for various diseases.

When should you use it?

Until now, it has been used successfully as an anti-inflammatory for treating rheumatic diseases such as arthritis and other inflammatory conditions such as gout. It is also used to treat diarrhea.

But today, there is great interest in its powerful antioxidant activity and especially in its proven ability to increase the body's defenses, so that it is not only useful for treating viral or bacterial infections, but it is being researched for its beneficial role in treating certain malignant tumors and leukemia. It is also useful as a supplement to lessen the adverse side effects of chemotherapy.

Presentation

In our country, it is mainly used in capsules and tablets that have an indicated dosage amount. Although it is not very common, it is also possible to find its dried bark, ready for preparing decoctions.

Remedies

BY ITSELF

Decoction: mix 2 table-spoons (30 grams) of dry cat's claw per 2 cups (0.5 liter) of water. Boil it for 15 to 20 minutes and let it steep for 5 minutes. Strain it and drink ¼ cup (60 milliliters) every 24 hours, preferably after meals.

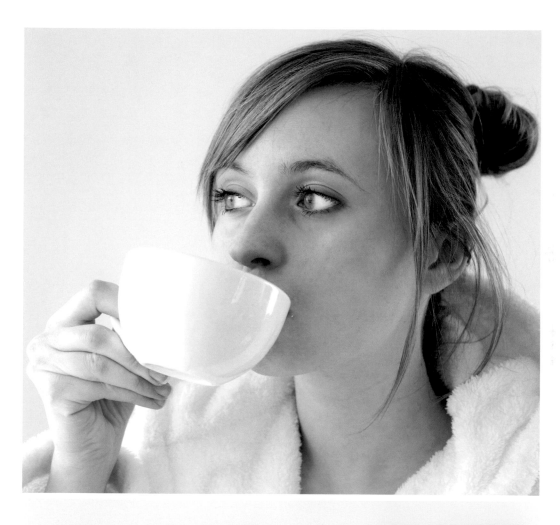

Precautions

It is contraindicated for persons suffering from peptic ulcer or gastritis, and during pregnancy and lactation.

Description

It is a climbing or sometimes creeping vine that grows to over 130 feet (40 meters) long and 65 feet (20 meters) high. Its opposite and oval leaves are simple. It has tiny and fine hairs (tomenta), and its tiny flowers grow in clusters.

Cultivation

It grows in South American forests where there is plenty of sunlight.

Harvesting

The bark of the roots and leaves are harvested by trained people.

Composition

It contains alkaloids, flavonoids, tannins, triterpenes, and steroids.

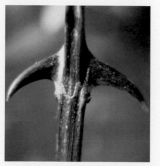

Clove

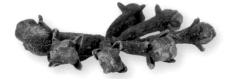

(Cariophylis aromaticus)

Calms toothaches

It is native to the Maluku Islands, and its name derives from its resemblance to a carpenter's nail. This spice has an intense aroma and a slightly spicy flavor, as well as some important medicinal virtues that were already known in ancient times: it is antiseptic and strengthens the stomach, so the plant became a treatment for pest epidemics. Its essential oil gives it its properties and fragrance. Today, it is used for manufacturing perfumes and cosmetics and as an analgesic in dentistry.

When should you use it?

It is a general stimulant, it increases appetite, and it has carminative effect (eliminates intestinal gas). But what stands out above all is its effective oral analgesic and antiseptic effect. In fact, its essential oil is used as a disinfectant, and therefore as an ingredient in toothpastes and mouthwashes, and it is used in antiseptic preparations that dentists use. When it is used externally, it also has anti-rheumatic effect.

Presentation

It is most often available as a spice, whole or in powder, although it is also possible to find its tincture and essential oil. Its essential oil is sold separately or as an ingredient in oral antiseptics and soothing medications for toothaches.

Remedies

BY ITSELF
Apply a clove directly to the affected area to quickly relieve toothache.

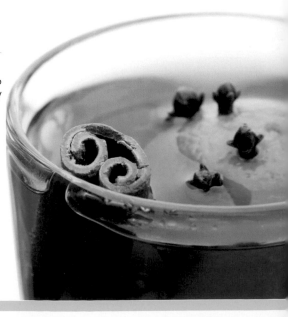

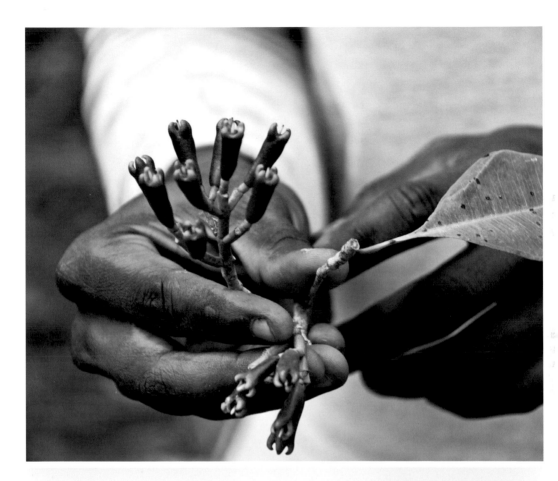

Precautions

It is contraindicated during pregnancy and lactation, and for persons suffering from gastritis and peptic ulcer.

Description

It is a tree of medium or large size that grows to 49 feet (15 meters) high. Its oval leaves are leathery, and its flowers (buds) are what create the spice.

Cultivation

It is native to the Maluku Islands in Indonesia, but now it is cultivated in many tropical countries.

Harvesting

Its flower buds are harvested when they begin to get a pink hue; they then become brown after undergoing a drying process. They can be kept in tightly closed glass jars inside a closet.

Composition

It contains essential oil, tannins, flavonoids, sterols, and triterpenes.

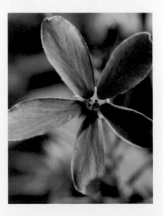

Eyebright

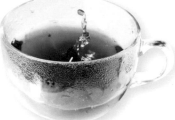

(Euphrasia officinalis)

Effective and safe eye drops

During the Middle Ages, eyebright was thought to have the power to heal "evil eye," and it was even described as a source of "precious water that clarifies man's vision" because it was used to rinse out swollen eyes.

When should you use it?

It has antiseptic, anti-inflammatory, and astringent properties that are especially effective for the conjunctival mucosa. It is a traditional remedy for conjunctivitis, blepharitis (inflammation of the eyelids), and watery eyes. It works very well when it is applied in poultices on styes and for the overall treatment of eye fatigue and disorders of the eye muscle or nerves. It is also good for rinsing out rheum because it clears up eye secretions, reduces inflammation, and decongests the conjunctiva. Also, when used for gargles, it fights coughing and hoarseness.

Presentation

Most often, it is available in troches (dried and ground), ready for making tea (½ teaspoon [2 to 3 grams] per cup of water) or decoctions. It is also possible to find it as an ingredient in homeopathic eye drops, which are very practical and totally harmless.

Remedies

BY ITSELF

Eye rinse: boil 1 ½ teaspoons of eyebright in a cup of water, for a couple of minutes. Let it steep for 10 minutes and strain. This eye rinse can be done 3 to 4 times a day. This decoction is exclusively for external use, so it can also be used to apply it as a compress. Similarly, it can be used for gargling and rinsing the mouth.

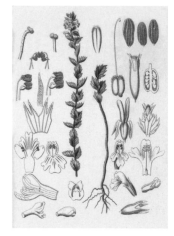

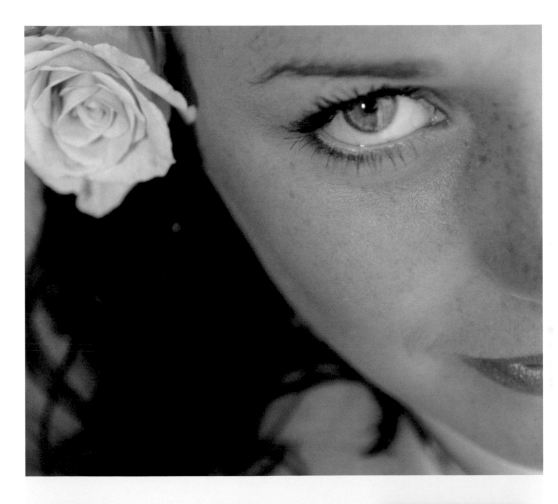

● Precautions
This plant has no contraindications or adverse side effects.

● Description
It is an annual plant that grows 4 to 12 inches (10 to 30 centimeters) high. The flowers are white with violet streaks, and two lips form its corolla. It parasitizes the roots of other plants.

● Cultivation
It grows in meadows and mountain forests throughout Europe. It is also naturalized in the American continent.

● Harvesting
The entire plant is harvested in summer, then it is dried quickly in the shade, because its essential oils degrade very easily. It is stored in sealed glass containers, away from light and moisture.

● Composition
It contains iridoids, tannins, lignans, and flavonoids.

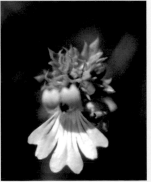

Sage

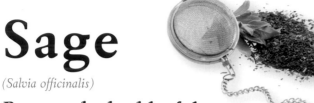

(Salvia officinalis)

Protects the health of the gums

Its name derives from the Latin salvare, meaning "to be saved," possibly in reference to the many medicinal virtues attributed to this popular plant. It is digestive, antiseptic, and a good ally for healthy hair, but it is also very valuable in the kitchen as an aromatic plant.

When should you use it?

Sage stimulates bile secretion, reduces the accumulation of intestinal gas, and calms abdominal cramps, so drinking sage tea after meals helps the digestive process. Sage also contains phytoestrogens, which have an estrogenic effect that alleviates hot flashes during menopause. Moreover, using it for gargles and mouthwashes helps soothe smoker's cough and itchy throat. It is a very useful treatment for gingivitis (gum inflammation) and canker sores, due to its anti-inflammatory, antiseptic, and astringent properties. It is also used for treating oily skin and revitalizing hair.

Presentation

It is very common to use its dried and chopped leaves for making tea (1 teaspoon per cup of water), in capsules filled with powdered plant (dosage is indicated by the manufacturer), in liquid extract (for internal use, ¼ to ½ teaspoon [1 to 3 milliliters] every 8 hours, and for external use, 1 teaspoon [5 milliliters] diluted in 1 cup [200 milliliters] of water several times a day), in tincture (for internal use, ½ to 1 ½ teaspoons [2.5 to 7.5 milliliters] every 8 hours), and essential oil (for external use, 2 to 3 drops in ½ cup [100 milliliters] several times a day).

Remedies

BY ITSELF
Sage infusion for gargling: boil ½ cup (100 milliliters) of water and turn off the heat when it starts boiling. Immediately add 2 teaspoons of sage. Stir it well, cover it, and let it steep for 10 minutes. Use this warm infusion for gargling several times a day.

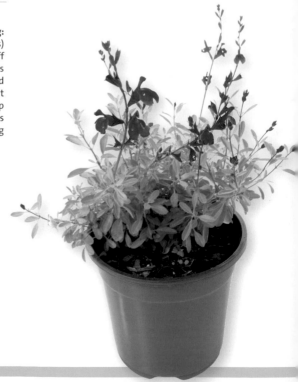

Insect bites

Sage is a useful antiseptic to soothe and heal insect bites in a simple and natural way. To reduce inflammation, apply a poultice made with juice from fresh crushed sage leaves. Place it on the bite until it dries. To relieve pain, apply a few drops of essential oil with a cotton swab.

Precautions

It is contraindicated for internal use during pregnancy and lactation.

Description

It is a shrub that can grow to 2 feet (70 centimeters) high. Its leaves have white undersides, and its purple, blue, or pink flowers grow clustered together in spikes.

Cultivation

It grows in chalky soil and adapts perfectly well to soil that is not very fertile near farm fields, ditches, and rocky slopes, generally in dry and sunny environments. It is very easy to grow in gardens or pots, using seeds or by planting cuttings.

Harvesting

The best time to harvest its leaves is in May. They are dried in the shade and stored in bags or boxes but never directly in glass or plastic jars.

Composition

It contains essential oil, flavonoids, tannins, and bitter substances.

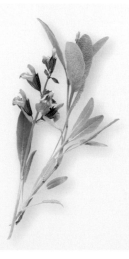

Plant index

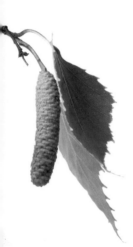

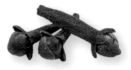

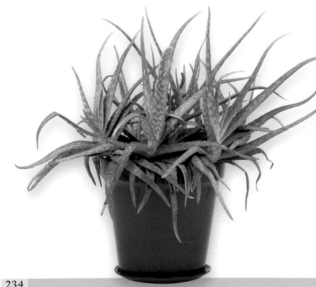

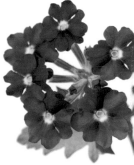

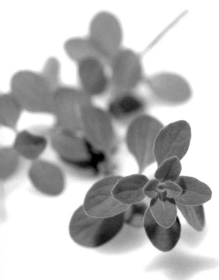

Glossary of terms

Adaptogen: it helps the body adapt to stress and physical exertion.

Analgesic: pain reliever.

Anesthetic: abolishes sensitivity to external stimuli.

Anthelmintic: destroys or helps expel intestinal parasites.

Anti-inflammatory: reduces inflammation.

Antibacterial: destroys or prevents the growth of bacteria.

Antibiotic: destroys or prevents the development of certain pathogenic microorganisms.

Anticoagulant: prevents blood clots.

Antiemetic: stops or prevents vomiting.

Antifungal: destroys or relieves fungal infections.

Antipyretic: effective against fever.

Antisclerotic: helps prevent or treats circulatory sclerosis.

Antiseptic: inhibits the development of pathogens that cause infection.

Antispasmodic: prevents or relieves involuntary muscle spasms.

Antitussive: suppresses cough.

Aphrodisiac: increases sexual potency and desire.

Appetite stimulant: stimulates the appetite.

Astringent: causes constriction and dryness in organic tissue, thus decreasing secretion.

Bronchodilator: dilates the bronchi.

Cardiotonic: has a tonic effect on the heart; increases force of contraction.

Carminative: prevents, alleviates, or expels gases from the digestive tract, relieving cramps and spasms.

Cholagogue: stimulates gallbladder contraction and increases bile flow.

Choleretic: stimulates bile production by the liver.

Cicatrizant: stimulates wound healing through scar formation.

Demulcent: softens and protects irritated or inflamed tissue.

Diaphoretic: stimulates sweating.

Digestive: aids digestion.

Diuretic: increases urine secretion and excretion.

Emetic: causes vomiting.

Emmenagogue: induces menstruation.

Emollient: moisturizes, softens, and protects the skin and mucous membranes.

Expectorant: helps to expel phlegm and mucous from the respiratory tract.

Extract: substance that is extracted from another in concentrated form and retains its properties.

Febrifuge: fever reducer.

Galactopoietic: promotes milk production.

Hemostatic: reduces bleeding and promotes clotting.

Hepatic: stimulates and promotes liver function.

Hypnotic: induces sleep.

Laxative: facilitates bowel movement.

Lipid-lowering: lowers blood cholesterol and/or triglycerides.

Lymphatic: tones and stimulates the lymphatic system.

Narcotics: produces stimulation or excitement followed by insensibility or stupor.

Pectoral: related to the chest. Agent for relieving disorders of the chest and lungs.

Purgative: causes emptying of the bowels.

Purifying: it purifies the blood or body.

Rubefacient: increases blood flow in the skin surface, causing redness.

Stimulant: increases stimulation through nervous tissue.

Stomatitis: inflammation of the mucous lining in the mouth.

Vasoconstrictor: causes contraction in the walls of the blood vessels.

Vasodilator: causes dilation of blood vessels.

Venotonic: promotes venous circulation.

Vermifuge: destroys intestinal parasites.

Vulnerary: promotes the healing of wounds, ulcers, or bruises.